Kratom

Countless Benefits That Come With the Use of Kratom

(A Comprehensive Guide on Things You Need to Know About Kratom)

Linette Gentry

Published By **Tyson Maxwell**

Linette Gentry

All Rights Reserved

Kratom: Countless Benefits That Come With the Use of Kratom (A Comprehensive Guide on Things You Need to Know About Kratom)

ISBN 978-1-998769-83-4

No part of this guidebook shall be reproduced in any form without permission in writing from the publisher except in the case of brief quotations embodied in critical articles or reviews.

Legal & Disclaimer

The information contained in this ebook is not designed to replace or take the place of any form of medicine or professional medical advice. The information in this ebook has been provided for educational & entertainment purposes only.

The information contained in this book has been compiled from sources deemed reliable, and it is accurate to the best of the Author's knowledge; however, the Author cannot guarantee its accuracy and validity and cannot be held liable for any errors or omissions. Changes are periodically made to this book. You must consult your doctor or get professional medical advice before using any of the suggested remedies, techniques, or information in this book.

Upon using the information contained in this book, you agree to hold harmless the Author from and against any damages, costs, and expenses, including any legal fees potentially resulting from the application of any of the information provided by this guide. This disclaimer applies to any damages or injury caused by the use and application, whether directly or indirectly, of any advice or information presented, whether for breach of contract, tort, negligence, personal injury, criminal intent, or under any other cause of action.

You agree to accept all risks of using the information presented inside this book. You need to consult a professional medical practitioner in order to ensure you are both able and healthy enough to participate in this program.

Table Of Contents

Chapter 1: KRATOM MIXED CONSUMPTION

General about mixed consumption

Mixed consumption is omnipresent and carries opportunities and risks. Thus, the simultaneous consumption of two or more psychotropic substances can lead to a completely new sensation, intensify, or mask an effect. On the other hand, interactions are possible that can adversely affect the experience or even make it dangerous.

Kratom mixed consumption with alcohol

Alcohol can intensify the effect of kratom and increase well-being. Especially the mixed consumption with beer, many reviews are dedicated. Accordingly, the beer gives the Kratomwirkung a new note. Even a small amount of beer can greatly influence the effect. In addition to strengthening the Kratomwirkung can also occur classic drowsiness that is otherwise known by alcohol. The two remedies seem to potentiate each other. After a certain amount of alcohol, the kratom effect is superimposed on that of the alcohol.

Overall, kratom works well with alcohol. There are no reports of negative interactions.

Kratom mixed-use with cannabis

The use of kratom, in combination with cannabis, is quite common and enjoys mostly positive feedback.

According to some reports, kratom covers the tired and sluggish effect of THC, due to the stimulating and activating effect of low-dose kratom. With increasing Kratomdosis, one is reinforcing the sedative properties of THC can not be excluded.

The positive mood of the kratom can give the consumption of cannabis a euphoric character. For example, some consumers use kratom to consume cannabis with positive well-being. Negative aspects of cannabis can be mitigated with kratom.

Furthermore, consumers report more intense intoxication and other facets of cannabis use when they also consume kratom.

Some consumers report from different angles and can specifically name the influence of kratom.

Dangerous Kratom mixed-use

MAOIs

MAO inhibitors are known as antidepressants, among others, and are more commonly used in cases of depression.

The mixed-use of kratom with so-called MAO inhibitors should be avoided. MAO inhibitors are substances that are present in medicines or natural products and can cause dangerous interactions with psychotropic substances.

They inhibit the enzyme monoamine oxidase, which degrades biogenic amines. The breakdown of psychoactive substances is inhibited by MAO inhibitors and thus prolongs or intensifies the effect. The increased burden on the body can pose risks and should definitely be avoided.

The combination of kratom and MAO inhibitors can prolong the effects as well as cause dangerous side effects. Therefore, it is advised to refrain from mixed consumption.

Dangerous interactions with other substances

The mixed consumption with the following substances should be avoided at all costs:

modafinil

Carisoprodol

Datura stramonium

propylhexedrine

THE ACTIVE INGREDIENTS

Kratom in its usual dosage form: Powder.

Kratom is a natural product and contains several psychoactive substances that are responsible for the kratomtypische effect in their entirety. Primarily, the so-called alkaloids are attributed to the mind-altering properties. Kratom comprises about 40 of these structurally related alkaloids.

Among others, the following compounds are contained in the kratom:

7-Hydroxymitragynin

ajmaline

Corynanthedin

Mitragynine

mitraphylline

Mitraversin

Payananthein

and more

The two most important active ingredients are mitragynine and 7-hydroxy mitragynine. They are structurally related to psilocybin and act as an agonist on the μ-opioid receptor, explaining the sedative effect of kratom.

Mitragynine represents about two-thirds of the alkaloid mixture. Overall, the alkaloid concentration in a Kratomblatt is about 0.5 %.

Mitragynine is not water-soluble and can go into solution in ordinary organic solvents such as acetone, methanol, ethanol, acetic acid, or diethyl ether. In pure form, mitragynine is present as a solid crystal and melts between 102 ° C and 106 ° C.

The fact that not one substance is responsible for the effect, but a mixture of various structurally related molecules. This is especially important when producing extracts or extracts.

KRATOM AS A PAINKILLER

Ordinary painkillers

Common over-the-counter analgesics are often ineffective or have serious side effects.

Aspirin may be cited as an example, it may be harmful to the gastrointestinal tract, and the blood-thinning effect may have further consequences.

Metamizole, a powerful prescription non-opioid analgesic, sometimes attacks the spinal cord.

Painkillers in the form of opiates have, in addition to side effects on addiction, although they are just the first choice for chronic pain but are given due to the risk of addiction only reluctant.

Kratom as an alternative

Kratom is a natural psychotropic drug with an analgesic effect. Kratom

is mostly present in Western Europe as a powdered sheet and can be purchased legally in online shops.

It is usually used as a relaxing natural drug that boosts mood and, depending on the dose, has a relaxing or euphoric effect.

Where does kratom come from?

The medical history of kratom dates back to the 19th century in Thailand. However, in addition to the analgesic effect, kratom also has other medical applications.

Thus kratom is used as a natural remedy for diarrhea. Likewise, it helps opiate addicts to escape their dependency while using kratom as a substitute. In Southeast Asia, kratom was also consumed by workers, who became less sensitive to the intense sunlight, making their daily work more bearable.

Due to its appetite-suppressing effect, it serves as a purely herbal weight-loss aid in Asia. This use should be discouraged.

ANALGESIC EFFECT OF KRATOM

The analgesic effect of kratom is comparable to that of codeine. The antinociceptive effect of 7-hydroxy mitragynine (one of the alkaloids of the kratom) is 13 times that of morphine (formerly morphine). Under antinociceptive effect is meant specifically the effect that counteracts the perception of pain. Kratom is, therefore, a very potent analgesic without the numerous and dangerous side effects of substances such as morphine, which also includes cross-tolerance.

The mechanism of action of kratom is the same as in opiates, which is reflected in similar effects and side effects.

With chronic daily use, it should be taken into account that addiction can develop.

As with all medications, kratom has dangerous interactions with other substances. Mixed-use of the following medicines should be avoided:

modafinil

Carisoprodol

Datura stramonium

propylhexedrine

DEALING WITH KRATOM AS A PAINKILLER

In general, especially for natural substances, the effective dose may depend very much on various factors. The sobriety of the stomach and body weight alone does not make it possible to estimate the right dose. Therefore, it is very good to start with small dosages. This will help develop a sense of kratom and provide a personalized dose without the inconvenience of overdose. These are often expressed by headaches or nausea, similar to a hangover known from alcohol. The remedy in such a case provides plenty of hydration, food, and lying down.

Daily consumption should be avoided. There are two good reasons for this: On the one hand, a tolerance quickly develops, which is reflected in increasing dosages, and on the other hand, there is an increased risk of developing an addiction.

Possible side effects besides the analgesic effect

Kratom is a psychotropic herbal natural drug. Thus, psychological effects can occur, such as a feeling of relaxation, contentment, or happiness. Depending on the dosage, it can cause a euphoric or relaxing effect.

PHARMACOLOGY

Depending on the variety, kratom contains a varying mixture of psychotropic alkaloids, which are responsible for the typical effects of kratom. Since the composition is thus subject to natural fluctuations, a pharmacological characterization is difficult.

The effect of kratom largely depends on the dose consumed. This paradoxical spectrum of action can not be fully explained pharmacologically, especially since very few studies on the effect of kratom have been carried out.

The sedative effect at higher doses is primarily due to the alkaloids mitragynine and 7-hydroxy mitragynine. These act as agonists on the μ-opioid receptors, in which opiates also interact. This explains the analogy to the effect of opiates.

In the stimulating effect is unclear how the mechanism of action works. Mitragynine and 7-hydroxy mitragynine are believed to favor delta-opioid receptors in low doses.

Animal studies have found that the cough-suppressing and analgesic effect of mitragynine is comparable to that of codeine. Here, the analgesic, so the pain-relieving effect, is many times more pronounced than that of morphine (formerly: morphine).

In mice, a cross-tolerance to morphine was found.

The mixed consumption of kratom with other psychotropic substances can cause serious side effects result. The combination of amphetamine, cocaine, or high doses of caffeine can induce high blood pressure. A combination with, for example, opiates or alcohol can lead to over-calming of the nervous system and, thus, to respiratory distress. Furthermore, mixing with MAO inhibitors should be avoided as this may affect and / or prolong the effect.

DEPENDENCE AND ADDICTIVE POTENTIAL

The topic of addictive potential also plays a major role in natural drugs such as kratom. Especially for first-time consumers, it is advisable to familiarize yourself with potential risks. The term "addiction" in this context stands for mental and physical dependence.

The area of addiction and dependency is barely explored for kratom, and there are few concrete reports from consumers who identify themselves as addicted or addicted.

Consumers who use kratom to relieve chronic pain can become physically dependent on daily consumption. A high frequency of use (daily or more often) and high dosages favor the development of an addiction.

First and foremost, kratom is a natural drug that enhances the well-being of the consumer and thus has addictive potential. In general, we humans tend to want to experience beautiful experiences again (addiction finally comes from searching). So it is with the kratom. The perceived effect would be caused again; the feeling is again be investigated. It is not so much a physical desire as a desire to increase his well-being again. This desire we know from everything that makes happy, including food, sports, sweets, or a hobby.

Since kratom can be perfectly integrated into everyday life, there is a risk that consumers will become a habit. The consumer gets used to the effect, and the intake becomes an integral part of everyday life. This habit can follow a mental dependence, which is associated with withdrawal symptoms at weaning. The abrupt withdrawal of kratom may cause discomfort or mild depression. The body may respond with withdrawal symptoms in the form of common flu-like symptoms as well as fatigue, insomnia, fatigue, or muscle aches.

Long-term consumers report a physical withdrawal of about one week and describe it as more pleasant than, for example, with caffeine withdrawal.

Another addictive potential arises when kratom is consumed to avoid grief, stress, bad mood, or general malaise. Kratom has a calming effect in such situations and unfolds its usual effect. This may result in kratom being abused as a way out of unpleasant moods.

The problem with long-term consumption is the formation of tolerance. If kratom is repeated and consumed in short periods of time, it can lead to the development of tolerance. The amount of kratom required for the usual effect is steadily increasing. As a result, consumption becomes more and more unpleasant and more expensive due to the increase in volumes. As the dose increases, physical stress increases, and health risk increases.

Chapter 2: WHAT ARE KRATOM EXTRACTS?

Kratom extracts are composed of Kratom in a highly concentrated form. They are usually made by infusing the Kratom leaves chopped or powdered for long periods of time. In this way, as much water as possible is evaporated, and a pasty, dense, and dark substance is obtained, which contains a high concentration of the plant's main active compounds.

These extracts can still be processed to create powders, liquid dyes, oils, or solid substances such as resin. As with any other plant extract, the purpose of producing kratom extract is to obtain a refined product that contains the main ingredients of the plant and can be taken in smaller but more concentrated doses.

High-quality kratom extracts are generally made by professional experts, who have already carried out various experiments with the plant and are familiar with the particular method for extracting its active ingredients.

HOW TO INTERPRET THE CLASSIFICATION OF EXTRACTS

Kratom extracts are usually classified as 1x, 5x, 10x, or other numbers followed by an "x." The meaning of this gradation is often misunderstood.

Many users believe that a kratom extract classified as 15x, for example, is 15 times more potent or contains 15 times more alkaloid than the normal untreated kratom leaves. This conception is wrong.

In fact, these gradations indicate the concentration factor of the extract based on the volume. For example, a 15x extract was obtained, starting from 15 grams of powdered kratom leaves and then reduced to produce 1 gram of concentrate. Similarly, a 4x extract was made starting from 4 grams and reducing them to 1.

Another widespread misconception is that extracts with a higher concentration rate are more powerful. For example, many people believe that 15x extracts are more powerful than 5x, for example.

However, this is not always true, essentially because the alkaloid content varies widely depending on the various types of kratom trees. Therefore, it is the variety of a kratom extract that indicates its intensity, and not the gradation, more precisely.

HOW TO USE KRATOM EXTRACTS

There is a vast controversy over kratom extracts and their safety. Some users claim that they increase the chances of tolerance and adverse effects. Just like any other substance, it all depends on common sense. After all, you wouldn't use a brazier with 85% hash oil if you had never smoked even a joint, right?

If it is the first time that you are consuming Kratom, it is always advisable to start with a non-concentrated product, such as chopped or powdered leaves. Try to choose a medium power variety, and start with a dose of 1-2 grams.

After becoming familiar with Kratom, you will understand the effects it has on yourself and your ideal dose. At this point, if you want to go further, you could try an extract to get more powerful effects by investing your money better.

When taking any kind of extract, the dosage is clearly essential. As we have previously observed, there is no real standard in the alkaloid content of the different kratom tree species. Therefore, it can be difficult to understand how much extract should be consumed to obtain the desired effects, reducing the negative effects as much as possible.

Below we give a very general estimate on how to proceed in the dosage of kratom extract: If you usually consume a dose of 2 grams of normal kratom powder, you can try 0.2-0.3 grams of 10x extract. If you are very upset about the adverse effects, you can take a lower dose, for example, 0.15 grams.

As mentioned previously, using kratom extracts is exactly like using any other concentrate. Follow your common sense and start with low dosages. After all, you will always have time to consume a little more if you need it, but you cannot cancel the dose if you start feeling side effects. Also, avoid taking the extracts too frequently, as you could develop a tolerance to Kratom.

THE EFFECTS OF KRATOM EXTRACTS

A high-quality kratom extract provides effects similar to normal kratom dust, but with smaller doses. Minimal doses of kratom cause relieving and stimulating sensations, comparable to those caused by amphetamine and cocaine.

Higher kratom doses, on the other hand, cause sedative effects similar to opium and other narcotics. Below is a general list of the effects caused by Kratom, both in powder and concentrated form.

Positive effects include:

- Stimulation

- Improved mood

- Greater ability to concentrate

- Strong relaxation

- Pain relief

- Sedative effects

- Increased sexual desire

Negative effects include:

- Nausea

- Vomiting

- Dry mouth

- Frequent urination

- Restlessness

- Tiredness and lack of coordination

- Fatigue

- Constipation

- Stomach pain

KRATOM CAPSULES

What are kratom capsules?

Kratom capsules are a great way to take kratom. Since the kratom is packed in gelatin capsules, the kratom taste can not spread in the mouth: the intake is thus "tasteless." This is a huge advantage over traditional forms of consumption, such as tea, juice, or yogurt.

Furthermore, in the manufacture of such capsules, little "residue" is produced. Kratom, which has not found its way into the capsule, collects in a plate and can be reused. It is no longer waste kratom, so in other forms of consumption. In the processing of several hundred grams, kratom is just as little wasted as the consumption of a few grams in the form of juice, tea, or kratom honey.

There is a downside; however: The effect may be delayed (experience 10-15 min), but there is no preparation time. After all, like so many things in life, it's a matter of taste.

How much fits in such a capsule?

A capsule size, " 00, " will fit around 440 mg (0.44 g to 480 mg (0.48 g).) Depending on how well you can swallow capsules, 5-6 capsules can be swallowed simultaneously. Of course, it varies from person to person.

This allows the consumer to take up to 3 g of kratom at a time with a sip of the beverage of choice. The capsule variant is thus suitable for small, as well as for larger amounts of the plant.

How do I make such capsules?

You can make capsules manually by filling the capsules " by hand." Unfortunately, this has some disadvantages:

it takes a long time

the kratom can not be compressed properly

Ultimately, only a small amount of kratom can be filled

That's why you take a capsule filler. These can already be bought at reasonable prices and are easy to handle. For example, 24 capsules can be filled at once. Furthermore, the kratom can be compressed well during filling. This is the only way to get 480 mg capsule size "00".

A capsule of size "00" costs about 1.5 cents and holds 480 mg.

How does a capsule filler work?

Essentially, such a capsule filler consists of 2 halves. In one comes the long end of the capsule, in the other the short one. In both halves, the capsules close off with the surface surrounded by an edge (which keeps the kratom in the filler).

Now spread kratom on the surface until all capsules are filled up. With a tamper, the kratom can now be compressed. Then the process is repeated.

Finally, both halves are brought together and compressed. The capsules are thus closed.

The small segment of the capsule is constructed so that it does not need to be filled. The kratom only comes into the long end of the capsule.

KRATOM BEGINNER GUIDE

The first use of kratom is particularly exciting for consumers who have had little or no experience with psychotropic substances.

requirements

For your first consumption, we recommend a day, afternoon, or evening when you are free of obligations and work. The effect may last for several hours and may end in sleep, depending on the dose. So you need time! The next day, it may come to a hangover, which is very similar to that of the alcohol. You should also consider this.

If you feel like it, invite a friend or other familiar person. This may take away the fear that you can share your feelings and feel safe. A Kratomer experience for two can lead to very interesting discussions.

Take the kratom on an empty stomach. In order to feel the effect of unmixed kratom in full intensity, you must take kratom on an empty stomach. Otherwise, the active ingredients are only very delayed in circulation, and the effect is subtle or not noticeable. Furthermore, the likelihood that you will feel worse decreases.

preparation

1. Inform yourself extensively about kratom!

2. Order the type of crumbs of your choice

3. Assign a precise balance; we recommend the following model:

Kratom works in the gram range. Even fractions of a gram may cause a noticeably different effect. For the Kratomkonsum, an ordinary kitchen scale is not enough.

Overdoses by estimating the amount may be felt in the form of nausea or a hangover the following day.

4. Choose a form of consumption and put everything you need ready.

If you do not want to get a capsule machine at the beginning, we recommend Kratomtee as a form of consumption. For that, you basically only need tea bags (we recommend peppermint) and a sweetener (honey or stevia). You probably will not taste it, but it is prepared quickly, acts quickly, and additionally hydrates your body.

5. Weigh one dose. You should note the following points:

Start with small amounts. The effective dose may vary considerably from person to person and can not be estimated on the basis of body weight or the like. In addition, kratom has a range of paradoxical activities. In low doses, it has an activating and euphoric effect, calming and relaxing in high doses.

So you can adjust yourself to an effect even with smaller dosages. "Much helps a lot" is not true here!

Concerning the dose: As a rough guideline, for example, Kratom Maeng Da Thai Pimps to be 1.5 - 2.5 g. This is a very potent strain and can cause a noticeable effect even at low dosages. In general, we recommend rather start with little and slowly refill.

6. Take the kratom to you. Do not give yourself too much time so that as many alkaloids as possible are taken into the circulation at the same time.

KRATOM HONEY

There are many ways to consume kratom. In addition to mixing with drinks or mixing with food, there is still a very simple and fast method. The preparation of kratom honey.

What are the disadvantages of ordinary kratom forms of consumption?

A disadvantage of the usual forms of consumption is, for example, the duration of the preparation. Thus, the preparation of a Kratom tea takes about 20-25 minutes. Although kratom tea can also simmer unattended, it takes a lot of time.

Another point is that taking kratom with the help of other ingredients is more expensive. It is quite possible that, for example, the orange juice as a medium exceeds the value of the actual kratom. This is, of course, only a small item but deserves to be mentioned.

The taste of kratom tea or kratom blended in orange juice is not exactly comfortable for many. It may take a while for the prepared drink to be drunk.

What is Kratom, honey?

Kratom honey is a paste made of kratom and honey, as the name suggests. The honey serves as a " binder " and binds the Kratompulver to a homogeneous paste. The honey fulfills several tasks and has other advantages:

The honey binds the hard-to-consume powder into a homogeneous mass.

The sweetness of the honey covers the intrinsic taste of kratom.

Honey is cheap. A bottle of liquid honey is enough for many applications.

Often liquid honey is already in the house.

The paste can be dosed well with a spoon.

Even larger amounts of kratom can be taken without much liquid or food.

What makes Kratom honey so interesting as a form of consumption?

The advantage of kratom honey is that the kratom is merely bound. For this reason, you only have to take a very small volume for you. The form of consumption is thus very effective and fast. Depending on the dosage, your kratom is consumed in no time.

How do I prepare Kratom honey?

Weigh out the appropriate amount of kratom and place it in a shallow cup or small bowl.

Add liquid honey. About as much volume as your kratom takes.

Stir the ingredients into a paste and adjust the amount of honey if necessary.

Take the paste to you. It is most pleasant to swallow the kratom honey directly with some water. Depending on how well this works, you can adjust the portion size.

Toss & Wash

In addition to the classic forms of consumption such as kratom tea or kratom capsules, there are also one of the other exotics such as kratom honey. Toss & Wash is just as rare, but also enjoys a good reputation among many consumers. In addition to the full range of effects, simple preparation is appreciated. In addition, Toss & Wash is perfectly tasteless when properly carried out. An experienced consumer has one of the most effective forms of consumption known.

If done incorrectly, Toss & Wash may cause kratom to be inhaled into the pharynx! The method requires some practice and should be done wisely.

What is the basic idea behind Toss & Wash?

Basically, at Toss & Wash, the kratom is swallowed with water so that it does not come into contact with the taste buds. In addition to capsules, it is one of the very few methods by which kratom can be taken tasteless. Instead of a capsule, a layer of water separates the kratom from the taste buds.

How does Toss & Wash work now?

Have a glass of water and the dose of kratom ready

Take a small sip of water in your mouth and make it to a pond

Tilt the head slightly backward (stuck up)

Hold the air! Otherwise, your kratom spreads in the mouth and throat

Place the kratom carefully and in the middle of the pond

Put on your glass and rinse the kratom down with the remaining water

Is it really that easy? Yes and no. More on this in the next paragraph.

What to look for

The water temperature plays a role in two ways. On the one hand, cold water stuns the taste sensation; on the other hand, warm water can be better swallowed. The right temperature is best found out by yourself.

You can practice with small amounts of kratom. Divide your Kratomdosis into many small single doses.

Of course, you should place the kratom as carefully as possible on the pond.

When done correctly, the method is tasteless, fast, and needs only a very manageable preparation. Consumers who have problems with the taste of kratom could find an alternative to the capsules in Toss & Wash.

Kratom in fruit juice

Kratom is well-known for its characteristic natural taste, and the question always arises as to how kratom can be consumed most pleasantly and quickly.

Orange juice is a medium for kratom

(with dissolved kratom the juice turns green)

Generally, we recommend ordering kratom in powder form. The surface-to-volume ratio falls in favor of the effect and simplifies the intake noticeably! Finally, a larger surface area ensures faster absorption of the active ingredients.

Particularly important in the choice of the form of consumption is that it does not distort or limit the effect of alkaloids. For example, taking extended beyond food the absorption of the active ingredients and weakens under certain circumstances, the effect of kratom from.

For this reason, the intake with liquid offers. The kratom powder can be " dissolved " and then ingested. As an alternative to the fruit juice, kratom tea can also be prepared.

Kratom powder can be easily stirred into fruit juice. A milk frother is a helpful tool. Thus, the powder can be dissolved homogeneously in the fruit juice, which greatly improves the taste. Due to its mass, kratom powder quickly settles to the bottom of the vessel, so it is advisable to stir once before each sip. Depending on the taste, the ratio of juice to powder can be adjusted.

As a juice, orange juice offers, as the acidity and sweetness well covered the Kratomeigengeschmack. This form of intake is perceived as particularly pleasant.

Grapefruit juice is not recommended for beginners since grapefruit contains active ingredients that can greatly alter the effect and duration of kratom consumption.

Kratom tea

General information on the oral intake of kratom

Traditionally, kratom is taken orally and rarely smoked. The uptake of the psychotropic agents of the cataract is most effective through the digestive tract. Already in the 19th century, fresh kratom leaves were chewed in Southeast Asia for medical purposes.

If kratom leaves or Kratompulver are consumed, all contained psychotropic alkaloids completely in the circulation, and the entire spectrum of action of the cretaceous plant can be effective.

If, on the other hand, only the active ingredients are extracted, depending on the solvent, it can lead to some alkaloids not being dissolved or only partially dissolved. When using such an extract, not all active ingredients may enter the circulation, and the spectrum of action of the cratome is not completely available.

The classic among the forms of consumption: the kratom tea

Probably the most common form of consumption of kratom is kratom tea. The principle of Kratom tea differs only slightly from the preparation of an ordinary herbal tea.

The basis is powdered kratom or kratom leaves.

Further notes on the preparation of a Kratom tea

Extraction: The effect of the kratom tea varies depending on whether the crumb powder or the kratom leaves are screened off or not. It is unlikely that all active ingredients will be completely dissolved. If the leaves or powder are removed before consumption, the full range of effects may not be available.

Adding acid: The alkaloids present in the kratom can be better dissolved in an acidic environment. The addition of, for example, citric acid increases the mass of dissolved active ingredients.

Sugar & Honey: Since kratom is inherently bitter in taste, adding sugar or honey can significantly enhance the taste of the tea.

Temperature: If the kratom tea is still consumed while it is warm, this can accelerate the absorption of the active ingredient in the circulation. The circuit can absorb active ingredients faster if they already have a higher temperature than, for example, room or refrigerator temperature. In general, the solubility of substances is strongly dependent on the temperature.

Sober stomach: The condition of the stomach exerts a major influence on the effects of orally administered kratom. Shortly after a meal, the intake of alkaloids is severely limited. The likelihood increases that the active ingredients are absorbed so slowly in the circulation that no effect is perceived. There is simply no effect. However, when the stomach is empty, the alkaloids can be absorbed without hindrance.

Stir often: This concerns the preparation of Kratom tea with the help of Kratompulver, which is consumed with. The crumb powder is the pulverized leaf of the crumb tree. It is, therefore, not a substance that can go into solution in the classical sense, such as salt or sugar. The Kratompulver will thus settle overtime at the bottom of the cup or glass. It is therefore advisable to stir once before each sip so that no sediment forms.

KRATOM SORT

General

Kratom is a herbal product, so there are several different varieties with noticeable fluctuations in drug concentrations. Kratom is growing not only in the country of origin in

Thailand but also in neighboring states of Southeast Asia.

As with other plant species, it is common in kratom to breed new and more potent varieties. For example, the dominant strain " Maeng Da Thai Pimps " was created. It is a very potent strain, which enjoys great popularity for this reason. Even a relatively small dosage can cause noticeable psychological effects.

Furthermore, the varieties are labeled with names such as "Bali," "Thai," or "Maeng Da." She does not necessarily have anything to do with the country of origin; for example, "Thai" is no longer grown in Thailand.

Not only the effect varies depending on the variety, but also side effects, and the respective dose depends on the choice of the leaf. It is recommended to buy different types to find the right one for you.

Classification according to the leaf vein color

In addition to the classification of the varieties according to their origin, there is another: The leaf vein color. In the case of the cratoma, the leaf color says a lot about the contained drug concentration. For example, the leaves with white veins are considered to be more activating.

Generally, a distinction is made in three-leaf vein colors:

Red Vein (Red Vein)

Green Vein (Green Vein)

White Vein

The color of the vein allows conclusions to be drawn about the composition of the active ingredients and thus the effect. This is a way of categorizing cratome types.

Which crumb types are available? A small selection.

Red vein - kratom variety with red leaf veins and a sedating character

Borneo Red

Bali Red

Green vein - kratom variety with green leaf veins and balanced character

Borneo Green

Malay Green

Bali Green

White vein - kratom variety with white leaf veins and activating character

Borneo White

Sumatra White

Bali white

KRATOM MAENG DA

The variety of Maeng Da is considered one of the most potent varieties and is therefore highly popular.

Varieties such as Maeng Da Thai Pimps are not varieties in the sense that they are derived from a specific tree species but represent a mixture of several varieties dar. The variety mentioned consists, for example, of about 6 to 10 Kratomsorten and is very stable in quality.

The fact that several varieties are mixed results in averaging of the alkaloid concentrations. If the concentration of an alkaloid in harvest is weaker, it can be intercepted by another variety.

By mixing several varieties, it comes to a balanced Alkaloidgehalt and thus to a characteristic effect that stands out from individual varieties.

The quality of the variety hardly fluctuates and therefore enjoys great popularity.

"Maeng Da" stands for " improved " quality and thus emphasizes the particularly intense effect. The most common is the variety of Maeng Da Thai Pimps, it is considered the most potent and is constantly recommended.

KRATOM MAENG DA EFFECT

The main effects may be stimulation, happiness, and reassurance. Lower doses may be more stimulant, while at higher dosages, dreamy, sedative effects may be more emphasized. In addition, kratom is often also attributed to an aphrodisiac effect.

Of the different varieties, kratom from Thailand can have the strongest energetic effect. Maeng Da can be considered as a high-quality Thai variety and, as such, is the strongest available variety.

The effect occurs within 10 minutes and lasts for several hours.

WARNING

Not intended for persons under 18 years.

The effect depends on a number of factors, such as body weight, time of ingestion (before or after eating), and general mood.

We advise against driving under the influence of Kratom car or undertake other activities that require full concentration. The use of kratom in high dosages can lead to a mild addiction. Common side effects include loss of appetite, dry mouth, and constipation. Prolonged use can lead to insomnia, skin discoloration (mainly on the cheeks) and weight loss. Do not combine with MAO inhibitors.

MAENG DA PREPARATION

There are several ways to consume kratom. Traditionally, the leaves are grated and eaten, followed by drinking warm water, tea, or coffee. The kratom powder can also be taken in a milkshake with honey as a flavoring supplement. The leaves can also be drunk or extracted as tea. The resin extract is made by boiling a water extract until residues are left, which can be formed into a small ball.

The effect

The effect of the variety Kratom Maeng Da is described as stimulating and intense. It is strong and potent compared to other varieties. Furthermore, the analgesic effect of this variety should be above average. The drug concentration appears to be distributed so that the stimulating and euphoric effect is in the foreground.

dosage

Since it is a very strong strain, only a small dose is needed to produce a psychic effect.

In general, it is difficult for plant products to make a statement about the correct dosage. For potent varieties like Maeng Da, it is, therefore, advisable to start with small doses. It also depends on whether tolerance has already been developed — for example, the consumption of other cratoms or opiates.

Maeng Da Thai Pimps Dosage (rough orientation)

Desired effectbeginner

euphorisierend2.5 g - 3.5 g

Balanced3.5 g - 5.5 g

sedating5.5 g upwards

The variety of Kratom Maeng Da Thai Pimps is usually slightly more expensive than other cratoms. However, this price difference is offset by increased drug concentration. Consumers report noticeably more intensive effects and are happy to recommend the variety despite the increased price.

In general, it is worth ordering large quantities of kratom as the price per kilogram drops significantly. It should also be noted that, usually, several revenues are needed to find the right dosage. So should be ordered per variety to be tested at least a quantity of about 20g. This corresponds to about 3 to 4 different dosages.

KRATOM MINDANAO GREEN

Mindanao is a type of crater with green leaf veins.

The variety comes from the Philippine island of Mindanao. Mindanao is the second-largest island in the Philippines. It is also the southernmost archipelago. More information about the island

If you are a little more familiar with customs, you will notice that we have a special variety here. Usually, kratom comes from Malaysia or Indonesia. The Philippines is a rather unusual site for kratom and shows different vegetation than the usual cultivation. For this reason, a different alkaloid distribution can be expected.

The effect of Mindanao can be very clearly classified in the spectrum of greens. The variety shows an opioid component as well as an activating character.

It is noticeable that the effect of some consumers has an above-average psychological effect, which manifests itself in well-being and a brighter mood.

The strength is described as above average and should be considered at the first dose.

In terms of price, the Mindanao Kratom is located in the upper midfield. In view of the strength, one can speak of a very good price-performance ratio.

The availability is good; only the orderable quantities are lower. The largest package size offered is 250 g.

If you do not want a strong sedative effect but do not want to do without the psychic component, Mindanao is very good for you.

KRATOM THAI

The variety of Thai is considered one of the strongest Kratomsorten available. Originally the variety comes from Thailand, as the name suggests. However, kratom has been banned in Thailand since 1943, and the Thai variety is now grown in other Asian countries.

This variety is suitable for increasing the well-being and the activity. The rising satisfaction and euphoria make everyday tasks easier to accomplish. The concentration is increased, and everything seems to be more productive and faster. Good motivational music can positively enhance the effect.

KRATOM MALAY

The variety Malay is usually a Green Vein variety and thus a combination of relaxing and stimulating effect. Malay has a relaxing effect, and concentration is increased. The effect is balanced and therefore ideal for activities where calm and concentration are important, for example, office work.

Kratom Bali

The variety of Bali acts sedating and relaxing at high dosages. The effect is most similar to that of opium. The variety is ideal for relaxing on the sofa or bed. Daydreams and a pleasant half-sleep can occur and give the consumer a few hours of rest and relaxation. Sedative varieties like Bali should rather be consumed in small groups or alone so that the effect can unfold.

Chapter 3: THE 9 POSITIVE EFFECTS OF KRATOM

1) Stimulating

The stimulating effects of kratom increase attention and physical energy. For some, the energy level was higher than they are used to, causing some nervousness. This can be reduced by drinking water and/or eating foods to dilute the stomach. The effects of kratom from low to medium dosages generally last 2-4 hours.

2) Improves the mood

Most customers point out that kratom works based on spirit and cognitive status. In low dosage, it can significantly reduce fatigue and create a feeling of mild euphoria. This can go so far that a deep sense of satisfaction and wellbeing can be achieved. In larger dosages, kratom can produce euphoric feelings. This is probably explained by the many alkaloids that stimulate opioid receptors in the brain.

3) Increases concentration and stamina

In small doses, kratom acts as a strong cup of coffee, but then better. Where the caffeine of a cup of coffee lasts only a short time, the effects of the kratom last much longer. For a few hours, it's an intense focus booster. People who work for hours can experience the benefits of concentration and stamina. Students will be able to get more attention to the courses, and professionals will be able to meet deadlines. The white and green varieties are particularly useful in purifying the mind and thinking hard.

4) Improves sleep

Consuming kratom at a higher dose can help people with (chronic) sleep problems. It closes the mind from daily worries and provides a complete, relaxed, deep sleep. Many clients state that improving sleep is precisely why they take kratom.

5) pain relief

People with (chronic) pain or physical discomfort can use kratom as an alternative supplement for prescription painkillers. It stimulates mu-opioid receptors to relieve temporary or chronic pain. To relieve physical discomforts such as headache/migraine, arthritis pain, vascular pain, muscle pain, or chronic pain. That rarely make a normal lifestyle possible. For some, kratom has offered the opportunity to rebuild their lives. As an analgesic, kratom is considered safer and less addictive than the most stronger medications currently prescribed by doctors.

6) Relax the body

The use of higher dosages has a calming effect on body and mind. Slower breathing and a lower heart rate are some of the beneficial effects of this herb. By relaxing your body, you can get rid of stressful thoughts. The effect of kratom reduces physical and / or mental tension and can also help reduce nervousness.

7) Supports overall health

Kratom has proven to be a powerful antioxidant containing various substances used to fight a variety of diseases. In addition, there are more than 40 different alkaloids that are isolated from kratom. Each contains antibacterial properties that can significantly boost the immune system.

(Caution: Always consult a doctor if you have a medical condition.)

8) Prolongs sexual performance

Some men use kratom to last longer during sexual intercourse. It is very useful for men who suffer from premature ejaculation. People who wrote a review on kratom indicated that 1 or 2 grams of regular crumb powder is enough to delay ejaculation significantly.

9) Increase your social skills

Do not worry while enjoying social interactions. Kratom can suppress social anxiety, which is helpful when meeting new people. It makes you social as a person, making it easier for you to speak in public. Social and friendly behavior can be exactly the reason for you to go out, enjoy life, and meet new people.

KRATOM VS. SALVIA

Kratom and Salvia divinorum are usually sold through ethnobotanical stores. Salvia reached incredible popularity a few decades ago, and for that reason, has also received negative media attention. The attention Salvia received resulted in many states in Europe and America that banished this legal substance. Kratom is now in the same direction as Salvia, just as popularity is rapidly increasing.

Kratom and Salvia are two completely different herbs. The main difference between Kratom and Salvia is that Salvia has psychedelic and hallucinogenic effects, and kratom does not. Maybe that's why kratom does not seem so attractive to young people looking for thrills to get high. Kratom does not create hallucinations and is naturally calming and euphoric by nature.

There are plenty of ways to experience hallucinations or euphoric experiences in the modern world, thanks to the liking of Kratom and Salvia. Common, naturally-derived substances such as Salvia and kratom provide a nonsynthetic window between serene, euphoric experiences. Indigenous people have used these herbs for many centuries. These substances have significantly different legal status and laws that apply within Europe, the US, and the globe to restrict consumption. Regardless of their legal status, kratom and Salvia are available in various forms worldwide.

Kratom

Kratom is a large tree found in the regions of Southeast Asia. Within Thailand, the tree is usually found all over the country, but mainly in the southern regions. Kratom contains many alkaloids, including mitraphylline, mitragynine, and 7-hydroxy mitragynine. Kratom is traditionally used by farmers and workers in Thailand and Malaysia to increase their productivity but also as a substitute for opium. Kratom is often used as a new psychoactive substance within the global market.

Kratombeschreibung

In Southeast Asia, kratom leaves are usually freshly distorted. The fresh leaves are usually chewed or used as a tea. Kratom leaves are rarely smoked because too much is needed for a joint or a pipe.

For shipping kratom in Europe and America, the leaves are lyophilized. Thereafter, they are cut into a powder form or ground. As long as it is airtight and stored in the dark, the dried coagulum powder can be preserved for up to six months.

The known effects of kratom

Low doses (5 grams) are reported to have stimulating effects (used to combat fatigue during long hours), while at low dosages, they have sedative-narcotic effects. Kratom is known to be relaxing and euphoric while providing a soothing and balanced experience.

Salvia divinorum

Salvia divinorum (fortune-teller sage) is a psychoactive plant of the mint family (Lamiaceae). Primeval in the forest regions in Oaxaca, Mexico. The plant is psychoactive and causes short but powerful hallucinations. For this reason, Salvia is traditionally used by the Mazatec Indians for medical purposes and religious practices.

Salvia divinorum is traditionally consumed by sucking or chewing the fresh leaves from a cigar-like roll or, alternatively, crushing the leaves to make a drinkable infusion or tea.

Salvia is mainly smoked in the West today. The smoking of these dry leaves is known to induce short, but strong hallucinations, and the effects of salvinorin A have often been compared to those of DOB or LSD. In addition, nebulizers are often used to inhale the salvia extract. An alternative method is to mix salvia powder with a bit of juice or tea, similar to juice.

The use of Salvia in the West as a new psychoactive substance dates back to the 1990s. In 2009, Salvia was identified as the substance most plant-based, and 2012, third, just behind kratom. This is also explained by the fact that Salvia and its active component 'Salvinorin A' are increasingly controlled in different countries under different regulatory frameworks.

Salviabeschreibung

Salvia divinorum is usually sold as leaves or seeds. But be warned, recent studies of products containing Salvia divinorum have shown a discrepancy between the label and the actual components of the products. Caffeine, vitamin E, and other unrelated items have been identified as adulterants within the product. It's wise to double-check it and order it from reliable sellers only.

Well-known effects of Salvia

Unlike kratom, Salvia has strong psychedelic effects on its users and often creates glowing hallucinations that can last over two or three minutes each time. Like other plant-based substances, there are often limited scientific studies among people showing chronic or acute toxicity associated with its use; nevertheless, clinical observations have shown long-lasting psychosis in vulnerable individuals. However, there are currently no data on deaths from the use of Salvia divinorum.

Kratom and Salvia Divinorum connect

It is highly recommended that both Kratom and Salvia should not be mixed. Users have reported a strong feeling of nausea and even heavy periods of vomiting. The combination of Kratom and Salvia is strictly discouraged!

These are two different herbs that have a completely different effect on the body and mind. The series of disease is thought to be triggered by the binding of two different opioid receptors together. Salvia is a k-opioid agonist, and kratom is known to be a mu-opioid agonist and a delta agonist; every k-opioid agonist blocks the mu and delta receptors, which more than likely causes a bad experience for the user.

THE CHEMISTRY OF KRATOM

Until recently, Kratom (Mitragyna speciose) was largely unknown in the West. In the few studies published, mitragynine was mentioned as the most active alkaloid in kratom. But what do we really know about this plant? It has been used by peoples in Asia for centuries and has been identified by Westerners only a century before. Here is a brief description of the chemical composition of kratom and the alkaloids found therein.

Kratom is an opiate agonist with an interesting pharmaceutical and chemical composition. It has strong anesthetic properties and is often used as a replacement for conventional opiates. In small doses, kratom has a stimulating effect, which translates into more energy, social skills, and improved mood. Similar to a cup of coffee and / or two beers. At a higher dose, kratom may have a sedative effect, leading to calming and sedating effects. Similar to powerful analgesics or opiates. (Boyer 2008)

Chemical structure of kratom

The effects of kratom can be traced to the powerful alkaloids found in the leaves of the plant. Most types of alkaloids in kratom are Yohimbe, Uncaria indoles, and Oxindole. These simple components interact with cells in the body and therefore stimulate the nervous system. According to our knowledge, there are at least 40 of these alkaloids that were actually found in kratom. (Shellard 1974 Shellard 1978) Some of the chemicals are:

Alkaloid profile of kratom

ALKALOIDSPERCENTAGEMEDICINAL

mitragynine66%analgesic,   antitussive, antidiarrheal, adrenergic, antimalarial

Paynantheine9%smooth muscle relaxer

Speciogynine7%smooth muscle relaxer

7-hydroxy   mitragynine2%analgesic, antitussive, antidiarrheal

Speciociliatine1%weak opioid agonist

Speciofoline<1%analgesic, antitussive

Isospeciofoline<1%

Mitraphylline<1%immunostimulant, anti-leukemic

Isomitraphylline<1%immunostimulant

Speciophylline<1%anti-leukemic

Mitrafoline<1%

Isomitrafoline<1%

Rhynchophylline<1%vasodilator, antihypertensive, calcium channel blocker, antiaggregant, anti-inflammatory, antipyretic, anti-arrhythmic, anthelmintic

Isorhynchophylline<1%immunostimulant

Ajmalicine<1%Cerebrocirculant, antiaggregant, anti-adrenergic, sedative, anticonvulsant, smooth muscle relaxer

Corynantheidine<1%opioid agonist

Corynoxeine<1%calcium channel blocker

Corynoxine<1%anti-locomotive

Corynoxins B<1%anti-locomotive

Mitragynine oxindole B<1%

Ciliaphylline<1%analgesic, antitussive

Mitraciliatine<1%

Research has shown that mitragynine and 7-hydroxymitragyn are the most important of all alkaloids isolated from kratom. These two are predominantly responsible for the analgesic, soothing, euphoric, and stimulant effects of kratom. They appear to be structurally similar to yohimbine alkaloids but do not have the same effect on body and mind. They produce, for example, no psychedelic side effects.

Although Mitragyna speciosa is by no means an opiate, both alkaloids act as opioid agonists in the body. It should be noted that the exact mechanism of kratom on the mind and body is far from certain. For a long time, it was believed that mitragynine was responsible for the action of the herb. New studies have shown, however, that 7-hydroxy mitragynine has a stronger effect on opioid receptors and is therefore mainly responsible for the narcotic effect. The opinion among botanists is divided, and this proves the complexity of the chemical composition of kratom.

Mitragynine

Mitragynine, chemical name $C_{23}H_{30}N_2O_4$, was first isolated by Hooper in 1907 and later added by Field in 1921. An average kratom plant contains at least 0.5% mitragynine (Iamshaman 2008), making it the most dominant alkaloid on the list above. Similar to the effects of Yohimbe alkaloids, mitragynine binds itself to the alpha

adrenoceptors in the cells of the body. Subsequent simulation of these postsynaptic adrenoceptors causes most of the effects we feel when we consume the plant.

Furthermore, it has been found that the stimulatory types of kratom (white and green) have a higher concentration of mitragynine compared to the red varieties of kratom. This could mean that mitragynine is responsible for the stimulant effect of kratom. Evidence of this is supported by scientific research. (Grewal 1932)

7-Hydroxymitragynin

7-hydroxy mitragynine, also known as $C_{23}H_{30}N_2O_5$, was discovered in 1993.

Especially the strong binding with Mu receptors is responsible for the "narcotic" feeling that is expressed (Matsumoto 2004). A striking difference between 7-hydroxy mitragynine and traditional opioids is that 7-hydroxy mitragynine does not induce hypoventilation (reduced supply of oxygen to the lungs), which eliminates the risk of asphyxiation, which is a high risk with traditional opioids.

KRATOM CONTROVERSY IN THE MEDIA

A new legal drug?

In the meantime, we have all heard of 'bath salt' and 'spice' in the media; Drugs that are easy to find and buy at your local gas station or tobacco shop. The Drug Enforcement Agency has recently cracked down on this variety of drug variations by labeling the main components as a controlled substance. The media are now targeting kratom, calling it the "latest legal drug wave."

However, it seems that, unfortunately, kratom has been dragged into this media hate without investigation. What the media intended to do is that substances like kratom are organic and have many healing benefits that have been used for decades.

The media and misunderstandings

When kratom is present in the media, it is often presented to us in a negative way and associated with harmful substances that kratom has nothing to do with. It is clear that kratom is still relatively unknown in the Western world. This seems to contribute to some common and unnecessary misunderstandings. Comparing kratom with opiates, as some journalists do, highlights abuse and addiction as somehow related to kratom, and the users of this gentle organic herb are carelessly and negatively stigmatized. That's why we show the most common misconceptions about kratom that have appeared in the media in recent months.

Wrong: Kratom is a substance of abuse

The consumption of kratom rarely leads to negative effects on the user. Kratom is not guilty of crimes. It certainly does not cause any aggressive behavior. It does not cause people to be affected and lose their inhibitions, like alcohol, for example. It does not pose a threat to society.

Kratom is not an alternative to street drugs. Although ignorant sellers also praise it to the market as such. Those who consume kratom as a "legal high" or hard drug substitute will be very disappointed. The users of kratom are often middle-aged and highly educated individuals who use it as an alternative to deal with anxiety, pain, depression, addictions, or other illnesses.

Wrong: Kratom is not safe.

If thousands of years of safe use are not considered sufficient proof to prove the safety of kratom, what then? Compared to many stimulants and prescription drugs, kratom is much safer. Kratom is known to contain a wide range of beneficial compounds, such as antioxidants and many more. Let us remember how many people have used kratom. How many incidents have been reported? That's right. No.

Wrong: Kratom is addictive

Kratom can become a habit for some, just like everything else. A kratom habit potentially plays in the same league as coffee. People drink coffee because they enjoy the caffeine boost. They enjoy it. They start to drink it more often. Continuous coffee consumption can accustom the user to drink it. It is natural that it might be difficult at first if they decide to give it up. This is similar to kratom and many other things in life.

Since the media often report negative allegations or assumptions about kratom, the real reasons why people use kratom are often completely ignored.

Kratom is a general stimulant and is an effective anti-anxiety drug. While it is not a long-term treatment, it can help in the short term and avoids various risks and side effects that include anti-depressants and anti-anxiety medications.

It is amazing that the Western media does not demonstrate a degree of openness to kratom, especially as a growing number of users clearly benefit from it.

IS KRATOM ADDICTIVE?

Kratom is not a drug, and therefore, it is not addictive.

Although a small number of people (mostly in Thailand) became dependent on kratom, kratom does not addict.

It is important to be responsible and not to take kratom on a daily basis. As with other substances such as alcohol, tobacco, coffee, etc., it is difficult to change habits with daily consumption.

For this reason, it is important not to use kratom on a daily basis!

Kratom is used to prevent withdrawal symptoms of drug addiction. That's because kratom works as a powerful painkiller at high dosages. Although kratom acts on opioid receptors, it is not an opiate itself and, therefore, it is not a dangerous drug like the known hard drugs.

In kratom, which is occasionally taken for recreational purposes, rather than every day, the possibility of habit-forming is excluded. Set your guidelines. In the beginning, do not experiment with kratom more than twice a month. Stop taking kratom immediately if you violate your guidelines.

THE STORY OF KRATOM

Apart from new and growing concerns about synthetic drugs, organically grown products have also been placed under close observation. That's why many false beliefs on natural products sprout up, and one of them is kratom. It is a natural herbal plant and is commonly used for its numerous therapeutic benefits.

Kratom is scientifically known as Mitragyna speciosa and is an original plant from countries in Southeast Asia such as Indonesia, Myanmar, Thailand, and Malaysia. The unique tree has an egg-shaped pointed shape with dark green and spherical yellow-flowered flowers. A crater tree can grow up to 15 meters and 5 meters wide (thickness). Kratom was first described in the 19th century by Pieter Willen Korthals, a Dutch botanist who came by ship from the Dutch East India Company (Dutch East India Company).

The herb is available in three different varieties: the whitish (white vein), the green-veined (Gree vein), and the red-veined (red vein). It is generally called Kratom, Ketum, Kakuam, Thom, Ithang, or Biak Biak in many parts of Southeast Asia and also in the Pacific Islands. Inhabitants of Thailand, Indonesia, and Malaysia, had used the plant extracts domestically before the West recognized its unique benefits in the 19th century. Kratom finished products are available in the form of fresh leaves, kratom extract, powdered kratom, kratom tincture, dried leaves, (liquid kratom), and kratom capsules.

Ban on kratom

Today, the sale and use of kratom have been banned in Malaysia, Myanmar, Thailand, Australia, New Zealand, Denmark, Latvia, Lithuania, Poland, and Sweden. Especially in Asian countries, individuals who own this herb are at risk of being arrested and prosecuted, which can even lead to imprisonment. In the rest of the world, the purchase and possession of kratom are allowed.

Kratom Thailand

Traditionally used by agricultural kratom workers in Thailand who chewed fresh kratom leaves to make their hard work more bearable. In 1939, Thailand became the first country to declare the sale and use of kratom a criminal act. The plant is classified as a "dangerous drug" and is in the same category as heroin and cocaine.

Kratom Malaysia

Malaysia declared kratom illegal in 2003, and in August 2014, the ban was extended to the sale and possession of fresh kratom leaves. In the same year, the authorities put together a four-day project that focused on putting an end to the cratoma markets in states such as Terengganu, Pahang, and Kelantan. This resulted in fifteen arrests and nearly 245 kilograms of kratom leaves and over eight hundred liters of prepared kratom tea (locally called "air ketum" - called kratom water).

The pressure was raised by Malaysian media, which linked kratom with dependency and abuse. The media reported abnormal use of kratom, in which kratom is mixed with tobacco and dried cow dung and then smoked, which would result in unpleasant effects. The following year, the Attorney General introduced policies to expand the ban and make kratom a criminal act. As a result, kratom has been re-classified and included in the list of "toxic substances" in the class of "dangerous drugs," making it even more illegal than the previous enforcement.

Kratom Australia

Australia is another country that recently declared kratom an illegal herb. During the discussions at the National Drugs and Poisons Schedule Committee in February 2003, Mitragyna speciosa was recognized as a toxic substance. Individual voices demonstrating his safety, harmlessness, and medical as well as therapeutic potential remained unheard. On January 1, 2005, the law came into force.

Kratom New Zealand

Notwithstanding being banned in New Zealand, New Zealand authorities have found that kratom has properties for opiate addiction. For a detoxification period of 6 weeks, individuals are allowed to use kratom against opiate withdrawal problems. Kratom has an effect on the same receptors that make the withdrawal symptoms more bearable. Within this period, the kratom dosage will gradually be reduced.

Kratom today

It is advisable to obtain your kratom products from a reliable seller who will give you the best advice. In an effort to make a distinction between real kratom and other harmful drugs, it is very important that you know how best to identify the plant. A lot of misleading information about kratom is in circulation, often far from the truth and misleading.

Despite its unique benefits, kratom should not be taken without consulting a doctor first. In particular, people with physical and / or mental symptoms are advised to see a doctor. Try natural methods only if nothing else helps.

For kratom products of high quality and expert advice, you are in the right place. Our people are very familiar with kratom and always ready to answer questions.

Chapter 4: 7 TIPS TO BUY KRATOM FROM TRUSTED KRATOM SELLERS

Thanks to the internet, we are able to acquire this particular product from Kratom vendors. Buy kratom online is usually 3 times (!) Cheaper than buying it from the local herbal or smart shop. As with online shopping, we recommend that you do some research before you buy kratom from a seller.

Do you want 100% natural kratom of the highest quality? Preferably as fresh as possible and also grown so that it lasts a long time? There are many stores that claim to have the freshest produce in the house. But how do you really know which is the best Kratom seller?

We offer you some practical tips.

1) legality

Before you even consider purchasing kratom from a seller, first make sure it's legal in your country or state.

2) value for money

The price of kratom depends on the quality, the season, the harvesting method, and the country of origin. Everyone, of course, loves low prices, but be sensible and stay away from dubious sellers selling outdated or bad merchandise. Only order from Kratom companies that adhere to high standards. "If anything is too good to be true, it usually is."

There is no general price system for kratom, so prices vary enormously. Do your homework. In most cases, the most popular sites offer the best deals. Often these sites have additional offers in their newsletter or social media.

3) Wide range of Kratom products

The most serious sellers offer a comprehensive range of Kratom products. Pay attention to the keywords of the Mitragyna speciosa plant. For example, the difference between Kratom Red Vein, Kratom White Vein, and Kratom Green Vein.

Does a kratom vendor offer (legitimate) herbs next to the kratom? If the shop devotes itself to so-called "legal drugs," it should be avoided. These are often smart or head shops that sell bad (processed) products that are supposedly 'high.' They offer poor quality kratom for a very high price.

Most Kratom sellers offer Kratom trial packs. By ordering them, you can try different products at reasonable prices. This will give you the opportunity to discover if kratom is valuable to you.

4) Safe (payment) environment

Check "https" tokens on the page asking for information. There is a green token in your address browser line that symbolizes a secure SSL connection.

Does the Kratom seller have clear privacy policies? Is your data protected? Are there any third files involved?

5) Shipping and Warranty

Will parcels be shipped within 24 hours? How long does the mind need?

What are the returns policy of this seller? Read and understand how shipments and warranties are covered by the Kratom seller. Is there a satisfaction guarantee?

Many customers of Kratomgardens want to receive their packages discreetly. Only the name and address of the customer will be visible outside.

6) Customer service and contact

Does the kratom seller have an office in the European Union? From where is the shipment made? Shipping outside the EU can lead to long delays, and import duties may apply.

Is it possible to contact the seller? Do you have a phone number or chat service to answer any questions?

7) Customer reviews

Read the reviews of other customers. The more positive reviews, the better.

HOW TO PROPERLY STORE KRATOM

Kratom is rapidly becoming a valuable tool for psychonauts, and for a good reason. But how long is its power preserved? Where would it be more appropriate to store it?

The Kratom has begun to enjoy widespread recognition in the West only recently. Coming from more rural Thailand, this substance was mainly used to increase the energy of the laborers before a hard day's work. The boost of mental concentration and physical activity generated by a cup of Kratom tea were ideal for helping workers break the monotony of their jobs and regain their energy lost during a hard day in the scorching sun. This plant, which still grows in nature, is usually boiled in water and consumed as a tea, a recipe that

Thai people traditionally used for hundreds of years.

To date, it has proven to be able to give more boldness and liveliness to a more lively activity, but this does not mean that it is suitable for carrying out twelve-hour agricultural work.

The versatility of this plant is perhaps one of its most interesting features. A small dose stimulates and awakens the mind, while a higher calm and relax.

If you are willing to buy large quantities of Kratom, you should also know how to store them properly. The most important aspect of preserving Kratom is to keep all its power intact.

Here are the best ways to ensure that the power of Kratom maintains the same levels over long periods of time.

OXIDATION

Do not leave it in contact with air for too long, or the leaves may deteriorate. Kratom in contact with oxygen quickly undergoes a process called "cross-linking," which reduces the effects induced by the leaves. The best way to avoid this situation is to store Kratom in an airtight container. The ideal would be a vacuum bag, but not everyone has a vacuum machine. So, both a bag and a jar with airtight closure can work just as well.

TEMPERATURE

Although most people store Kratom in the refrigerator, this system is not entirely necessary. The main objective, in fact, is to keep Kratom cool and to do this, it is enough to have a cupboard or pantry in a cool place, where the degradation times of the alkaloids can be significantly reduced.

UV RAYS

Store Kratom in a dark place. Prolonged exposure to sunlight dissolves leaf compounds, making them much less powerful. Furthermore, UV rays also tend to increase the temperature, which, as mentioned above, accelerates the decomposition processes.

HUMIDITY

Kratom leaves can become fertile ground for molds when high humidity is maintained for too long. If you are in such a situation, look closely at any parts affected by the shape and discard them, as they may not be used safely.

The best way to combat mold is by storing Kratom in a sealed plastic bag, placed in a glass jar or container of any kind, and then stored in a cool place.

HOW TO PREVENT NAUSEA FROM KRATOM

Kratom can relieve pain, reduce depression and anxiety, and offer a boost of energy. However, a high dosage can produce side effects. Find out how to take this herb without negative consequences.

The Kratom can make you feel more energized and positive. In addition, it can also relax, relieve pain, and help balance sleep. However, Kratom can also produce nausea and dizziness, rather unpleasant sensations that no one would ever feel. Here are some ways to prevent nausea:

KNOW AND RESPECT THE DOSES

When taking too large amounts of Kratom, one can easily feel stomach pains. With lower doses, but still effective, the risks could be significantly reduced.

To get the dose that is compatible with you , starts by taking just one gram of Kratom and wait to see its effects. If you don't get the results you want, take another gram after 45 minutes. As soon as you are able to get the desired sensations, discontinue use. The following day, pick up where you stopped and repeat the increase in doses gradually, stopping again before feeling too strong.

Instead of doing it by eye, use a digital scale, so you know the exact amount you are about to take. Even after finding the optimal dose of Kratom, wait at least four hours before taking another, to avoid any feelings of nausea.

By changing supplier or variety, the power of Kratom can vary, requiring dosage changes to avoid any unwanted side effects. Until you have gained some experience, always try to use the same variety of Kratom and the same supply sources.

ANTI-ACID 30 MINUTES BEFORE, A LIGHT SNACK 30 MINUTES AFTER

The body absorbs kratom alkaloids better on an empty stomach; lack of digestive traffic increases bioavailability. However, Kratom is notorious for causing nausea. Consuming it on an empty stomach only amplifies this side effect. Consumers can avoid nausea by taking antacids 30 minutes before taking Kratom. These tablets help neutralize stomach acid, counter gastric disorders, and release gas build-up.

Be careful. Although antacids help relieve nausea, they are known to be kratom enhancers; in fact, they increase the effects of kratom alkaloids. It is a compromise that many kratom consumers willingly trigger.

It is advisable to eat a light snack 30 minutes after taking Kratom.

CREATING A TEA INSTEAD OF MIXING THE DUST IN WATER

By taking a powdered dose of Kratom directly mixed in water, you will be more likely to experience nausea than you might feel from drinking tea.

When taking Kratom in powder, all the components of the plant are ingested: chlorophyll, waxes, fibers, etc. These compounds do not necessarily contribute to the set of effects induced by Kratom but can cause nausea. When preparing a tea, however, most of these useless compounds are eliminated, but the more powerful alkaloids remain in solution. This is why Kratom tea is particularly indicated to reduce the risk of nausea.

If you can't help but mix Kratom powder directly into the water, use a smaller amount than is normally used to make tea.

ADD GINGER TO REDUCE AND PREVENT NAUSEA

Ginger is a natural spice renowned for its ability to reduce nausea and counteract some stomach ailments. Grind them a little and add them to Kratom powder to mix in water or to make tea. The taste will be a little spicy, but it will be much more pleasant than pure Kratom powder.

If you experience severe nausea after taking Kratom, try chewing a piece of fresh ginger, it may help you feel better. Crystallized ginger is the root processed in the form of candied fruit and can be more pleasant to ingest than the fresh and spicy version, which is not appreciated by some.

Don't forget that even Cannabis is renowned for its ability to reduce nausea, just like ginger. If you are lucky enough to live in a country that has legalized this plant, you may have access to a completely natural remedy. However, don't forget that this will also bring an extra psychoactive boost to the herbal cocktail. Therefore, adopt this suggestion with due precautions.

By taking the necessary precautions and respecting the properties of Kratom, you will be able to get all the benefits of this beneficial herb without experiencing feelings of nausea or other unpleasant side effects.

IS KRATOM DETECTED BY A DRUG TEST?

For those facing a monthly drug test to keep their jobs, Kratom offers a relaxing (and untraceable) way to take a break on an idle Friday night.

Modern drug tests have improved as the list of accessible recreational drugs has expanded. Generally, these substances have existed for hundreds of years in their home country as stimulants or painkillers. The potential of some of these traditional self-medication remedies in the Western world has been fully realized.

It seems that Kratom started to be used as a light stimulant among Thai farmers and workers, who used the mental propulsion of this drug to find fun in an otherwise harsh and relentless life. Initially taken as a remedy for fatigue by the lower classes of Thailand hundreds of years ago, its medicinal properties were soon recognized, and Kraton quickly began to be used in the treatment of opium addiction, stomach problems, and, in some cases, like an aphrodisiac.

Kratom is generally sold in the form of tea leaves, powder, or capsules. It is consumed orally and has a mild psychoactive effect (it can excite and relax, depending on the dosage and the individual). A low dose of excites and concentrates the mind, and is often used to reduce pain, improve concentration and help promote a positive state of mind.

A high dosage induces a deep feeling of relaxation and tranquility and is useful for improving sleep quality, reducing stress, alleviating social anxiety, and treating opium addictions. The dosages are determined by the variety, as the strength of each variety varies greatly.

SO IS IT DETECTED BY AN ANTI-DROP TEST?

In short, no. Pure Kratom will not be detected in a standard drug test. A NIDA5 test (the most commonly used test) and also the 10-strip urine test will both be negative if you have only taken Kratom.

WHY IS IT NOT DETECTED?

The plant, Mmitragyna speciosa, does not have the same chemical composition as all the illicit drugs for which drug tests have been developed. The testers have no reason to look for this substance as it is completely legal.

Unless you live in Australia, Burma, Thailand, and Malaysia, there is nothing to worry about when you consume Kratom because it is 100% legal and considered an herbal remedy.

IS THERE ANY POSSIBILITY THAT IT WILL BE DETECTED BY AN ANTI-DRUG TEST?

No. The only thing that could definitively reveal the use of Kratom is a tailored test to find a specific residue of Mitragynine and its metabolite in urine, and it is highly unlikely to be faced with such a type of test. As mentioned above, since Kratom is legal almost everywhere, there is no reason to perform tests to detect this substance.

CAN IT CAPTAIN A FALSE POSITIVE?

Once again, no. It is not possible that Mitragynine and other alkaloids in Kratom can cause a false positive. It is much more likely that a false positive is produced by a drug or supplement taken before the test, so it is very important to tell the test person about any drug or supplement that you are taking. Ibuprofen and pseudoephedrine are well-known examples of drugs that can influence the outcome of the test. It has been documented that even eating a bagel with poppy seeds can, in some cases, give a positive result for opiates.

This demonstrates the sensitivity of such tests, but if Kratom is the only drug that is consumed, a false positive is incredibly unlikely. A second test would definitively prove that no drug was taken.

So the next time you feel controlled by the restrictive hands of the monthly drug test, instead of fantasizing about something you can't take, think about relaxing with a nice hot cup of Kratom tea. The effect will be quiet, relaxing, and above all, untraceable.

DOES KRATOM NO LONGER EFFECT?

Does Kratom No longer Effect? Here's How to Solve the Problem

Here are some practical tips for not getting used to Kratom.

Whether it's consumption for recreational or therapeutic purposes, Kratom has become a real phenomenon in the United States and Europe in recent years.

WHAT IS KRATOM?

Kratom is the name commonly used to refer to the dried leaves of a tropical deciduous tree, the Mitragyna speciosa. This member of the same coffee plant family is native to several Southeast Asian countries, particularly Thailand and Indonesia. It was used by indigenous peoples for centuries as a medicine, an herb with psychoactive and recreational properties, capable also of stimulating the body. Traditionally, fresh leaves were chewed by Thai workers as a real stimulant, to withstand the harsh rhythms of physical work better and to lift the mind in more monotonous activities.

HOW DOES KRATOM WORK?

Kratom contains more than 25 different active compounds, including the alkaloids Raubasina, Corinanteidina, Epicatechina, Mitrafillina, and Mitraginina pseudoindoxyl. The main active alkaloids are Mitragynine and 7-Hydroxymitraginine.

These latter alkaloids are both agonists of opioid and adrenergic receptors. At low doses, they act as a stimulant, inducing mainly adrenergic effects. At higher doses, sedatives prevail instead. The different varieties of Kratom induce variable effects depending on the alkaloid profile of each subspecies.

AT KRATOM

Especially in regular consumers, Kratom can be addictive. Just like any other substance, the body tends to get used to its consumption, reaching a certain tolerance to its effects. Progressively, this organ adapts its chemical compounds to compensate for the introduction of other external substances, with the aim of maintaining certain balances and homeostasis. This process translates into consumers in the form of addiction.

Addiction can push a person to increase the dosages to get the desired effects, moving away from what could instead be considered a light and reasonable daily dose. This tendency, with the passage of time, can lead to desensitization and abuse, creating, in some cases, forms of dependence.

What to do if Kratom no longer works? There are no magic and infallible solutions to avoid addiction from Kratom. However, some useful tips can be followed.

ALTERNATE THE DIFFERENT VARIETIES

The key is to avoid the "stagnant variety syndrome." This condition occurs when the same species of Kratom is taken for prolonged periods. Taking the same variety or the same mixture of subspecies every day, the body tends to show resistance to that substance in a much shorter time. It is therefore advisable to have several varieties of Kratom and mix them regularly, adjusting the dosages and alternating the varieties. In this way, the levels of agonism should not reach stable concentrations in the brain, and it will be more difficult for an addiction to occur.

MAKE A PAUSE

For those who have already experienced an addictive condition, the only solution is to take a break, so as to allow the brain to rest and restore the balance lost.

Reduce to a quarter the dose you were used to or even stop taking it for a few days. The longer the time between hiring will be, the faster the addiction will disappear.

To restore highly addictive situations, refrain from taking Kratom for at least 2 monthsAfter so much abstinence you will soon have no more addiction problems. If it does happen, then it will be advisable not to use Kratom for longer periods, in order to restore the original condition.

UNEXPECTED CONSUMERS

First of all, when taking Kratom, one must avoid creating an addictive situation. If you use Kratom as part of natural therapy for your personal health, try to limit the dosages to only once a day. It is always better to take a larger dose than many smaller ones. If you are interested in a recreational experience, try taking it only two or three times a week. In this way, your body will have enough time to regulate brain chemistry to its original levels, avoiding, in most cases, any addiction.

People who try it for the first time should take it as a powder, avoiding concentrates. The doses of the latter, in fact, could be too high and, consequently, the brain could adapt quickly to their action, generating addiction in a few days.

COFFEE & KRATOM: AN ENERGIZING MORNING MIX

Upgrade your morning drink with Kratom to get the best morning energy mix.

The Kratom, a relative of the coffee plant, is becoming increasingly popular. Many love Kratom for its energetic and uplifting effect but also for relaxing when taken at a low dosage. At higher doses, Kratom has a sedative and calming effect, with no adverse effects.

Given the increasing popularity of Kratom, it is natural that some people have discovered how to combine Kratom with other substances. Since Kratom is linked to coffee, it didn't take long before people started taking them together after discovering the wonderful synergy of Kratom with coffee.

Let's look at the benefits of taking Kratom along with your morning drink.

MIX OUT KRATOM AND COFFEE

Many of us can not start the day without one or two cups of coffee. We like coffee for its energizing effect because it can make us tired in the morning or in the afternoon. Some people have noticed that kratom and coffee have almost the same taste and begin to wonder if coffee can be replaced by kratom. Others do not like giving up their daily cup of coffee, although they agree with kratom and its effects. It was not long before someone associated them.

However, the mixture of coffee and kratom is really interesting considering their stimulating effect and their mutual influence.

DIFFERENCE BETWEEN COFFEE AND KRATOM

If you drink too much coffee, you know that it can be quite uncomfortable. You may feel a sense of "nervousness," start to sweat and feel excited. The "effect" of coffee can also be quite short. There is a boost of energy, but it can drop quickly, so you can feel even less energetic than before: you will have the formidable "fallout of coffee."

When taken in low doses, kratom increases energy levels and relaxes at the same time. There is no relapse like with coffee. Taking more kratom will be even more relaxing and soothing, likewise to taking opiates, but without the negative effects.

Adding kratom with coffee is a very good way to increase and improve their positive effects. You can add kratom to coffee for a stronger and more sustainable energy charge than coffee. You do not have to worry about nervousness or other unpleasant effects, such as drinking a lot of coffee.

HOW TO PREPARE COFFEE FOR KRATOM

Adding Kratom powder to your infusion is easy. There are instant mixtures of kratom that dissolve in water and are ideal for this purpose. You can simply put a teaspoon in the coffee, mix, and enjoy.

Others use a coffee machine or a French coffee maker to prepare their mixture of kratom and coffee. Add a teaspoon of kratom powder to your ground coffee and prepare it as usual.

If you have kratom leaves, you can then prepare a kratom tea to mix with coffee. Boil a cup of water. Take about 10-15 grams of kratom leaves per cup and pour it into boiling water. Boil the mixture on low heat for 15 minutes. Then filter the mixture with a coffee filter or a clean towel. Kratom tea can be mixed with coffee.

Regarding taste, adding sugar or cream is a good way to soften the slightly bitter taste of kratom, as in the case of black coffee.

If you add kratom to your morning coffee, you can enjoy the best of both worlds! You can enjoy the benefits of kratom as well as the benefits of coffee. When you mix kratom with your favorite coffee, you can create an excellent mix of energy for the start of the day!

How to make delicious Kratom tea

Kratom is a natural remedy that is increasingly successful because of its energizing and relaxing effect, depending on the type of food consumed. Kratom is a very versatile powder product that can be used in many different ways. One of the most relaxing and enjoyable moments is to take it in the form of tea. Here is the recipe.

BUT BEFORE SOME SHORT CONSIDERATIONS

First, we would like to say that kratom (called mitragynine), unlike other alkaloids found in other plant species, is resistant to high temperatures. This means that the risk of losing efficiency when it comes to a hot water solution is minimal. However, we recommend that you do not cook it too long.

Adding the juice of a whole lemon will give you an even more delicious drink. This gives not only more taste, but the acid contained in the juice also better protects the alkaloids of kratom.

KRATOM DOSE

The amount of kratom you can add to your tea depends on the type of effect you want to feel. This plant can affect humans differently. You will then need to calculate the dose that best suits your needs. In this context, we present the following table, which could be useful as a starting point:

1 gram: Very light effects

3 grams: Effects contained

5 grams: Standard dose for those who consume Kratom

10 grams: Very strong effects

> 11 grams: Extremely strong effects. Only people who have experience with this substance can venture here.

HOW TO MAKE KRATOM TEA

It is very easy to make Kratom tea. In order to proceed, you will need to get:

A small saucepan with a spout

A filter or paper filter for coffee

water

Kratom in powder

1 lemon

Optional: honey, sugar, cinnamon, or any other ingredient that can bring the flavor you like best.

PREPARATION

Pour 1½ cup of water into the saucepan and squeeze the lemon inside.

Bring water to a boil and add Kratom powder in the dosage most appropriate to your needs.

Mix everything and let the water continue to boil for about 15 minutes.

Remove the pan from the heat.

Place the strainer over the cup and slowly pour the Kratom tea. In this way, you should collect all those residues present in the powder, making sure you get a transparent and sediment-free tea.

You can now add anything that can tease your palate.

Good fun!

Note: Dust accumulated in the filter can be collected and reused. You will get a lighter tea, but you will have the chance to recycle it. If not, you can throw it away.

Chapter 5: WHAT ARE THE SYMPTOMS OF ENJOYMENT POSTUMES CAUSED BY KRATOM?

Although these substances are entirely different, kratom hangover is very similar to alcohol.

Difficulty falling asleep and waking up

It has been shown that some kratom varieties have sedative properties. This would explain why one of the side effects sleep deeper and longer. Some people may appreciate this effect, which is considered one of the least problematic symptoms of kratom hangover. However, you can feel pretty good when you wake up, and it's never pleasant.

a headache.

An illness from kratom is not comparable to the usual headache. It is a malaise that tends to concentrate around the base of the skull / upper neck. It is a tension in the cervix that is usually caused by the most stimulating varieties. In other cases, you may experience normal headaches with tormenting and stabbing pains in the top and front of the head (which you have often tried after an alcoholic night). This last form of migraine is due to dehydration.

nausea

Nausea indicates that your body has received an excessive amount of kratom. Fortunately, nausea caused by the kratom hangover is fairly mild and does not cause too much discomfort.

AVOIDING CRATOMIC DAMAGE

Hangover Kratom can occur for a variety of reasons. Most commonly, dehydration occurs.

Some scientific evidence confirms that kratom dehydrates the body. The best way to avoid kratom hangover is to drink lots of water. In this way, you can minimize the effects described above.

Obviously, your body also has the tolerance to kratom, and you need to be able to handle its cans properly. Although it is normal to make many trials and mistakes before finding the right dosage, one must always try to know its limits. In addition, we advise everyone to eat well and exercise during exercise. This helps to reduce other potential factors that could contribute to the hangover. The most essential thing is not to forget, to hydrate, and never to go beyond the limits. It takes more than the tolerance of your body can be a risky and dangerous exercise.

KRATOM IS A NATURAL PAINTER: SPORT TRAINING, INTENSE PHYSICAL WORK -

For serious and chronic diseases.

When the pain is a constant or frequent partner, and the body can no longer handle synthetic painkillers. Or get used to it, and you'll have to look for a replacement - a new painkiller that will also relieve pain but have less impact on the entire body. In such cases, look for natural painkillers, the most popular being opium. But opium has one, two, its major disadvantages: Opium quickly causes addiction and is illegal. Here you should pay attention to kratom!

During intensive sports training.

To achieve good results, you need to increase more, jump higher, "I can not go through" ... All achievements and sporting results at a high level are sweaty and painful! And the pain stays with the athlete not only during the training but also afterward. This is why among professional athletes, especially in Asia, in recent decades and in the Western Hemisphere, as a natural analgesic.

With painful physical work.

For this reason, humanity is beginning to use kratom to relieve their physical suffering. Challenging living conditions and strenuous physical labor have forced farmers in Thailand, Malaysia, Indonesia, and a number of other Southeast Asian countries where kratom is growing to seek ... resources and sources to lighten their livelihood to "get up tomorrow", Since then, people started chewing kratom leaves, then brewing kratom, smoking ...

The Benefits of Kratom Compared to Other Painkillers?

Natural product - an alternative to artificial drugs.

It is sold by law in cities, including the United States.

It costs less than opiates and many synthetic painkillers.

For example, it has minor side effects compared to the same opium.

Virtually no dependency when used wisely.

If you need to get rid of the pain and are already taking or not taking any artificial painkillers, try kratom, an effective natural pain reliever.

WHAT ARE ENTHEOGENS?

We know a whole range of plants that can be considered as entheogenic bacteria - some are more popular, others less so. Popular entheogens are a variety of teas, from black and classic green to exotic old pubs and ethnic mats. The very popular coffee is also a kind of entheogen - we drink it vigorously. Cocoa beans are also an entheogen!

And here are some of the most exotic entheogens known to a small group of consumers, but which are not prevented from having much stronger or more exciting properties than the popular coffee, cocoa,

116

and tea mentioned above. Is> Kratom, Leuzea, Guarana, Ginko Biloba, Kola nut, Tribulus, Guayusa, Sagan Daili, Yohimbe, Tongkat Ali ... This list can c for a long time, and each plant has its merit for humanity.

Why are entheogens necessary?

As mentioned above, entheogens, affects the mental and physical state of a person. For example, millions of people around the world do not represent the beginning of their day without a cup of coffee: it tones, allows you to wake up, and goes into business. Kratom is another less known entheogen that relieves pain, helps you cope with strenuous work or physical training, improves your mood, and relieves depression ...

Each entheogen has special properties that, combined with the rational use of the drug, help a person to better express his abilities. It's stupid to neglect. Again, everything is within reasonable limits - chocolate coffee, tea, should not be abused.

117

The Application of entheogens

Each entheogen has its own methods of use and rules methods of use. We recommend that you examine them carefully before taking any medicine. And above all, always remember that the poison is toxic in small quantities, then in large quantities! This is applicable to everything in our lives. After all, even water, which we have 80%, you can die drinking a lot at a time! Remember this.

HOW TO USE KRATOM? - FUNCTIONS OF INCREASE IN DOSAGE, EFFECT, TONER

In general, kratom is used for:

is used for:

Increase the general tone of daily activities (both physically and mentally);

Physical training;

Overcoming odepression

As an analgesic for hard work and chronic diseases

118

Facilitate the release of drugs (especially opiates) and alcohol dependence.

Dosage and properties of kratom to increase tone

To stimulate mental and physical activity, it is often recommended to use 2 to 5 g (half a teaspoon per teaspoon with a blade) of kratom in one step. Also, kratom should not be taken more than once a day and no more than two or three times a week so that the stimulating effect does not disappear over time.

The green grades of kratom are better suited to raise the tone.

Use kratom to relieve pain:

One of the most popular features of kratom is the relief of pain caused by chronic diseases and the speed of physical work and exercise. Kratom is, in some cases, an excellent natural substitute for synthetic painkillers, which has always been proven. iIn this case, you should start taking kratom at the dose of 6 g and gradually bring it to 10-15 g if necessary. nIn some cases, you may need to carry large amounts of kratom.

Buy for the analgesic effect, especially varieties of red kratom.

The sedative effect of kratom

If you take 10 grams or more kratom, you can expect a pronounced relaxing effect. Perfect for a relaxing evening at home, listening to music, "restarting" after a busy day.

Dosage of Kratom for the relief of post narcotic syndrome.

Kratom has proven to be a natural alternative to chemicals that survive withdrawal syndrome (especially opiates) and even alcohol dependence. Of course, kratom does not have as much effect as a method, but for a well-intentioned person, it is a good substitute for plastics.

In this case, the dosage may range from 15 to 50 grams of kratom leaves, which have been comminuted 2 to 4 times per day during the first three days. On the fourth day and the following days, it is necessary to reduce the dose by increasing the well-being ...

And we emphasize again: In each case, it is necessary to choose the dose of kratom, starting with a smaller one, individually, until the desired effect is achieved.

KRATOM FOR LEISURE: RELAX, KEEP FORMS, EUPHORIA IN OUR LIFE

Kratom for recovery

Relaxation - steam bath and relaxation. Feel the warm waves of happiness that carry the body: you want to lie down, listen to relaxing music, or take a nap. It is best to use red kratom at 4 to 8 grams per person;

Enthusiastic - now we take less kratom (1 to 3 grams), but white or green color. Suitable for situations where you need to prepare for exams, create a robot that requires focus and attention, use it during a workout, or "recharge" after a sleepless night, make an excellent substitute for coffee;

The euphoria is a very interesting trait that is not accessible to everyone: 8-15 grams of kratom evoke joy, a feeling of lightness of the body, and the desire for a smile. It should be noted that the constant realization of such a condition is impossible - the break time of at least 3 weeks!

Try it out and make sure the effect is really unusual and always different from the previous one. Also, each variety has its own "notes" and some differences, depending on the variety (red, white, green, yellow) and the variety itself (Maeng Da, Kapuas, Bentuangie). Also, we can recommend the use of a particular variety and experience with the combination of green, red, and white varieties, find your cooking methods, and make sure that these holidays are remembered.

Remember that it is not recommended to use kratom daily! Otherwise, the beneficial effects of kratom will be minimized and disappear. The amount of infused tea increases. Also, none of the national websites provide information translated from English sources and personally reviewed by the site's authors. To maintain a new perception of kratom, it is recommended to alternate kratom species and varieties. First, each type has its characteristics and, secondly; each variety gives its atmosphere and its differences in the prevailing effects. White and green varieties are considered red energy-related. Although there are two components in each of the types. Green varieties are considered more versatile with balanced effects. Also, yellow varieties appear. A small amount provides vital energy, and an average large amount of tea leaves contain the necessary relaxation that will be useful in the evening after work of the day. Due to the unique composition of alkaloids, each variety has its characteristics. Some types provide relaxation and relaxation, others a concentration, and a charge of energy. At the same time, the analgesic properties of kratom may be expressed to varying degrees depending on the variety. Kratom helps in managing arthritis - pain, legs, and back - traumatic pain. Because of its combination of vitamins, alkaloids, and properties, kratom facilitates the progression of viral and respiratory diseases.

When making kratom tea, do not forget to keep your personal perception in mind, familiarize yourself with the minimum of tea leaves to choose the optimal portion adapted to your needs. An attentive and conscious attitude gives you the opportunity to obtain maximum benefits and pleasant sensations. For anxiety and panic attacks, it is possible to perform short-term treatment in small portions with interruptions of use of up to several days.

HEALING PROPERTIES OF KRATOM: ANALGESICS, ANTIDEPRESSANTS, REHABILITATION, RELIEF, TRANQUILIZERS

Important factors:

Mass - the higher the weight, the higher the kratom dosage is to achieve the desired effect;

Age - Over the years, people are more sensitive to the anesthetic and toning effects of kratom, their body becomes "disciplined", requiring a different amount of active ingredient to begin to relax.

Personal Predisposition - A dozen other factors determine your sensitivity to all alkaloids in kratom.

Only these indicators make the difference between the effects.

Medical properties

Since the 18th century, Thai and Malaysian doctors have been using kratom in their practice. There is evidence on this and reports from some European organizations.

Features of the application:

Sedative - a calming effect that drastically reduces anxiety and tension. It also shows patients contraindicated for standard sleeping pills.

Pain Relief - The analgesic effect of people with arthritis and osteoarthritis can be attributed to the specific action of kratom. This method of pain relief method provided that no other medication is used at the same time as kratom, which suppresses the respiratory and nervous centers.

Antidepressants: This effect has been discovered by psychologists in patients with prolonged depression. When used, 5-7 grams of Kratom improves mood; It should also be noted that kratom improves concentration, alertness and endurance while maintaining overall tone. In other words, you can say that you become very "sober".

Respiratory properties - This may seem unusual, but it is in this way that by eliminating pain, the agents diminish the sensitivity of the receptors responsible for intercostal muscle contraction and coughing. Therefore, kratom relieves the symptoms of cough, but does not cure - it is important to remember;

Rehabilitation for alcoholics and drug addicts - Facilitates withdrawal syndrome by acting on opioid receptors and helps to overcome the desire to continue to use alcohol and drugs.

Relief from tobacco addiction.

HOW TO IMPROVE THE EFFECT OF KRATOM TO BRING MAXIMUM BENEFIT?

Store the kratom in a cool place ,dark and dry. Kratom, like any other herbal medicine, loses its properties quickly. And at high humidity, kratom rots and becomes raw.

The best option is to keep the crumb powder in an airtight container in the erefrigerator. But if you have a little amount and do not want to "stretch out" the pleasure for months, a closed locker in the apartment, away from any heating, is well suited to keeping kratom. Store the powder in places that are inaccessible to children.

How to increase the effect of kratom during preparation and consumption.

The substances we need are not released immediately. The crater should, therefore, last a little longer - at least 20 minutes. And knead well.

The acidic environment is a catalyst - add lemon to the tea (not a slice but half a lemon), lime juice, grapefruit, orange ...

This highlights the taste of kratom,

Spices - The little turmeric, cinnamon, and other spices to taste will only enhance the effects of kratom. Some people drink kratom with coffee, mate ... Caffeine and thiamine are not suitable for kratom. It is, therefore, best not to mix kratom with regular tea and coffee and to separate consumption in a timely manner.

It would be better to drink a glass of freshly squeezed grapefruit juice 20 to 30 minutes before eating kratom - this contributes to better uptake of mitragynine, the main active ingredient of kratom.

Do not eat or consume kratom before and after meals so as not to dilute the absorption of the medicine.

An effective way to improve the effect of kratom is to heat it in a thermos. Hot (70-80 ° C), but no boiled water, pour the powder into a thermos. Add the lemon juice, honey or sugar and let rest for one and a half hours.

THE HEALING PROPERTIES OF KRATOM IN MEDICINE

Although zagain and mitragynine are chemically similar (they are indole derivatives) and interact with opioid receptors, their pharmacological effects vary considerably. If Zagain is typically used for a single dose, it can be used as a "substitution treatment" such as methadone.

The great advantage of kratom is that it has a legal status in most countries of the world. This is one of the safest ways to eliminate acute of the syndrome in patients.

It is the cheapest and safer alternative to methadone. There are currently numerous reports of successful use of kratom in detoxification, even in severe forms of opioid dependence. Also, people who have high hopes of using kratom in the treatment of self-treatment and addiction must understand that kratom, although potentially safe and effective in uncontrolled practices and long term, is hardly useful, on the contrary.

The efficient use of kratom in the treatment of acute and chronic pain syndrome, in the context of the use of "classic" opioid analgesics, is of great interest because it allows the reduction of doses of the latter while maintaining a high level. And an analgesic quality. In this case, there may also be a slowdown in the development of tolerance to morphine-related substances, which generally leads to a downturn in the physical dependence of these substances.

In addition to its psychotropic activity, kratom has a number of urgent properties, which are evoked by the presence of many other biologically active substances in the leaves. These include pronounced antioxidant substances, immunostimulatory properties with antibacterial, and antiviral effects as well as substances that influence the cardiovascular system. According to some sources, even on the anticancer properties of plants.

It is very effective to use kratom as an another option to codeine in various antitussives. In contrast to codeine and other opiates, kratom has a considerable advantage: it does not stop breathing; it helps to spit and does not prevent it. Also, we must not forget its antibacterial and immunostimulatory properties in the treatment of infectious diseases of the upper respiratory tract. These properties of kratom are also very useful in treating pain syndrome after certain surgical procedures, as this would reduce the risk of developing infectious complications in such cases. As for the efficacy of analgesia, kratom is roughly comparable to codeine and some of its derivatives, while leaf alkaloids, often called "opioid analgesics," dozens of times more massive than morphine, have shown rather unexpected results. In the early 1970s, pharmaceutical company Kline and the French pharmacological laboratory conducted an experiment with mitragynine, introducing an alkaloid isolated in humans.

In a personal letter addressed to Karl Jansen in 1986, Raffauf announced that this study had been discontinued due to acute and unacceptable side effects. He wrote: "It is likely that this phenomenon is caused by the pharmacological differences between isolated mitragynine and natural kratom leaves, which contain many other active alkaloids." Pure mitragynine causes nausea, vomiting, double vision, muscle problems, and side effects. Effects on the Cardiovascular System, Therefore, it can not, by default, be used as such under conditions analogous to a number of illicit drugs in the opium series, another important feature of kratom and its alkaloids.

In 1999, Pennapa Spcharon, director of the National Institute of Thai Traditional Medicine in Bangkok, concluded that kratom could be prescribed for patients with depression, but pointed out that this requires a lot of additional research, and any potential use of kratom in the treatment of drug addiction should be considered exclusively as part of the complex therapy.

Thus, if in ethnic medicine in many countries where the plant Mitragyna speciosa grows wild, all kinds of preparations of its leaves have been used successfully since ancient times by popular healers for a wide variety of pathologies and symptoms, official medicine Western is just starting to get used to this amazing plant.

Chapter 6: KRATOM - THE PROS AND CONS OR WHAT YOU NEED TO KNOW

Although this drug is controversial in several countries, more and more people are supporting the legality of kratom, and for reasons. In this article, we examine the pros and cons of kratom, for which this plant deserves the right of free sale, and what to consider when using kratom.

Advantages of kratom

The local population in Asia has been using kratom for centuries to improve their ability to work and relieve the pain of strenuous physical work and constant illness. Consider the importance of kratom in the modern world.

Kratom is a natural painkiller. Historically, kratom is used in hard physical work and in the modern world for sports training to relieve pain during and after hard work or heavy training. It is essential to note that kratom is a natural anesthetic and an excellent alternative to artificial painkillers for the treatment of serious diseases such as oncology, chronic pain, and performance improvement. In the East Asian homeland of kratom, workers and peasants have been chewing kratom leaves for hundreds, even thousands of years, while working hard and monotonous. In the modern world, the use of kratom has found many applications before intensive sports training.

Finish the hangover. Kratom helps fight hangover syndrome by positively improving the condition of the person. And also noticed a nuance, if you drink kratom, it attracts less alcohol.

Relief of the withdrawal of the drug.

Very often, kratom is used as a natural substitute for methadone when stopping opium use. Of course, natural kratom is not as effective as synthetic drugs, but it is less damaging to health and, if you prefer, "jump off" is an effective alternative.

Improve the mental state. With the moderate and rare use of kratom, there is a general improvement in the mental state of a person: the desire to live, to do something, a mood and an attitude towards others, is a depressed state leveled. This effect is not apparent (as in marijuana, for example), but the quality of mental life improves imperceptibly.

Kratom in sport. Many modern sports fans, especially in Asia, take kratom before training. This facilitates heavy and monotonous work with sports equipment or your body.

The beneficial effect of kratom on health. As some studies show (kratom is not helpful to conventional medicine), moderate administration improves cardiac function, normalizes blood pressure, stimulates blood vessels, and even lowers blood sugar. Everything is individual here, listen to your body.

The advantages of kratom are apparent: this natural product can undoubtedly be used to improve the quality of life as well as mental and physiological health. But like everything that happens in this world, kratom has "two sides of the coin" in case of abuse, another feature of kratom can be manifested.

Pity Kratom, what you need to know

Do not abuse kratom, take high doses (for this to work), or take kratom too often! This is the main thing you need to know if you decide to buy kratom. And therefore.

If you frequently take a kratom, its effect diminishes, and you need to increase the number of leaves (powder) steadily. With the daily use of kratom, the stimulating effect (increased efficiency and improved mood) can completely disappear. Kratom addiction is not more expressive than getting used to coffee, drinking a cup of coffee 2 to 3 times a week, invigorating it, and drinking coffee in buckets all the time, the effect is less noticeable. And even the coffee stops to revive. The body gets used to caffeine. And, secondly, the substances contained in the kratom leaves may not have time to get rid of by the body, and this does not affect very well the health affecting the liver, the painful thinness, blackening of the skin, disturbance of the home and Care. All this manifests individually.

Chapter 7: Opioid Abuse In the United States

Since the introduction of opioid painkillers such as Oxycontin, Vicodin, and Percocet in the 1990s, the usage of these medications has grown significantly. According to the Institute of Medicine's 2011 study, around 100,000,000 Americans suffer from chronic pain each year. Even though depression is undeniably real and affects many individuals every day, the long-term consequences of using opioids to treat it may be far more detrimental than simply coping with the disease on one's own.

Around 26 million to 34 million opioid users are estimated to be throughout the globe, with two million abusing prescription opioids and almost half a million abusing heroin, according to estimates. The number of prescriptions for opioid medicines has increased dramatically in recent years in the United States.

A little over 76 million opioid prescriptions were written in 1991, and by 2011, the total had increased to 219 million, nearly doubling from the previous year's total. In 2004, 145,000 prescription opioids were filled; by 2012, the number had increased to more than 306,000. This period saw an almost twofold increase in the number of emergency room visits due to prescription opiate addiction. Prescription opioid addiction accounted for 5 per cent of admissions in 1997, and it continues to account for 1 per cent now, a decade later.

In 1999, around 2,000 people died as a result of heroin overdoses, and approximately 4,000 people died as a result of opioid medications prescribed by physicians. By 2013, the number of heroin-related deaths had reached around 10,000, while the number of opioid-related deaths had reached almost 19,000. It is important to remember that the same characteristics that make opioids addictive also make them lethal in large doses.

In the same brain areas as heroin and morphine, they generate euphoric effects when snorted or injected, but they are considerably more potent when snorted or injected improperly.

Opioids are often considered pleasant and well-being-inducing by those who use them. They have a proclivity to relive this event over and over again in their minds.

There is also the issue of intolerance to contend with. In response to frequent usage, opioid potency decreases, and users are encouraged to raise the dose. This increases the feeling of well-being while also increasing the risk of addiction.

Despite the dire repercussions, some people succumb to addiction, while others can avoid it altogether. Addiction is described as the obsessive seeking and usage of substances regularly. Some researchers think that heredity accounts for around half of the diversity in risk factors, with other variables such as mental health, socioeconomic position, and stressors playing a larger influence on risk. Even though there has been much dispute about this, it appears that the increase in opioids has also increased heroin usage, particularly among younger individuals.

Because heroin is more readily available and less expensive than painkillers, heroin usage has skyrocketed across the United States in recent years. In many places, heroin is more readily available than marijuana. Between 2005 and 2006, there was a substantial increase in the number of heroin users in the United States.

Since heroin was still illegal and uncontrolled in 2012, it has the potential to be mixed with other narcotics, making it more difficult to overdose on the substance. In addition, when injected, users are at a higher risk of developing hepatitis, HIV, and other blood-borne illnesses, among other things.

According to several surveys and pain management clinics, opioid prescriptions for chronic pain account for more than 90 per cent of all prescriptions, while pain management clinics account for only a small portion of the overall prescription.

The majority of primary care patients who receive opioids from their main care physician were long-term users, and more than 60 per cent were prescribed two to three different opioids by various doctors, according to the National Institute of Health. According to the Centers for Disease Control and Prevention, around 80 per cent of individuals who get "low dosage" opioid prescriptions are nevertheless responsible for roughly 20 per cent of overdoses in the United States. Patients who get high-dose prescriptions from a single practitioner account for an extra 40% of all overdoses, according to the study.

According to the available data, long-acting opioids are not only more effective in controlling pain, but they are also less likely to be abused. More than 40 per cent of overdoses in the United States are caused by patients who see numerous doctors and manipulate them for medications, according to the CDC. Because so many people have been accustomed to it, the world appears to be becoming more conscious of the problem of quicker escalation to larger dosages of medication. More policymakers are paying attention to the problem and looking for ways to develop answers.

However, we must also pay attention to how to treat people who are already suffering from substance abuse disorders. Several recent research has found a link between opioid addiction and mortality in the United States.

Opioids And Their Effects On The Brain

For ages, cultures have cherished the feelings of pleasure and pain alleviation that opioids may offer them. It was only after the American Civil War that morphine was produced from opium poppies that it was used as primary therapy. After morphine became widely available, pharma firms developed a non-addictive alternative for it: a cough syrup known as heroin, which was a commercial failure for most of the twentieth century.

Prescription opioids, such as oxycodone and fentanyl, are widely available in both medicine cabinets and on the streets in the United States. Every year, more people die from opioid overdoses than from vehicle accidents in the United States, but to understand why this has happened, we must go inside the human mind.

Chapter 8: Nerves In The Brain (Neurons)

Typically, when opioids reach the brain, they bind to tiny receptors on the ends of nerve fibers known as Neurotransmitters, which allow them to function. They become active as a result of the chemical messengers. Opioid receptors work in the other direction. It is their job to prevent electric impulses from passing through nerve tissues, which are also known as neuronal tissue.

Opioids are effective in the treatment of pain. For example, persons who suffer from chronic back pain transmit pain signals to their brain continuously through their spine. Opioids work by calming the nerves, allowing them to relax and ease their discomfort.

There are three important opioid receptors, which are designated as Kappa, Delta, and Mu in the body of a person. Mu receptors are essential because they are responsible for nearly all of the effects of opiates in humans. Taking an excessive amount of this opioid off-switch results in addiction. It relieves pain, alleviates anxiety, and fills the mind with feelings of warmth and pleasure, among other things.

The Addiction to Opioids in the Human Brain

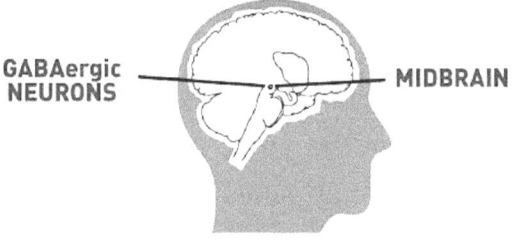

Mu-opiate receptors are found in the midbrain and are responsible for turning down GABAergic neurons, which results in addiction. Neurons in the midbrain are responsible for blocking the transfer of dopamine from other transmitters to the brain's   pleasure   circuits.

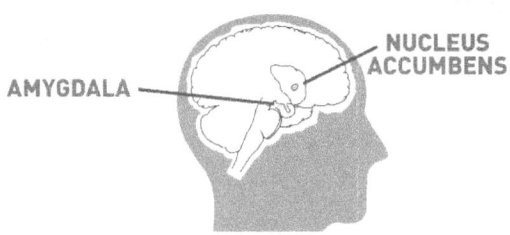

The nucleus accumbens (also known as the nucleus accumbens or NAc), which is located along with these pleasure circuits, releases a burst of dopamine, reinforcing the notion that opioid drug usage is pleasurable. The dopamine released by our fear center (the amygdala) reduces worry and tension, causing the decision-making centers of our brain to become overloaded and cravings to set in at the same time as a result of this.

The Opioid Pendulum And Addiction

Withdrawal is a side effect of all medicines that occurs when they are clearing the body; it is referred to as a dark side. After ingesting an excessive amount of beer or cocaine, you may suffer from a hangover the following day. Nonetheless, long-term opioids such as methadone do not alter an individual's outer behavior, since they can continue to drive and work.

Opioids progressively rewire the brain circuitry to a new normal state. Soon, addicts experience constant anxiety in the absence of opioids, and their stress hormones stay elevated.

Constipation and fluctuations in body temperature are common side effects of opioid usage; when the addictive drug is withdrawn, someone with opioid dependency will have persistent diarrhea, hot flushes, or goosebumps. Opioid withdrawal has been described as the sickest sensation a person has ever felt, and addiction is driven by a desperate need for relief.

A Synopsis of Kratom

Kratom is believed to have originated in Burma and Malaysia but has also been found in Thailand, Taiwan, and Burma. Around 1834, it was first reported by a Dutch botanist called Pieter Willem Karthus. Mitragyna Speciosa, he called the Kratom for the leaf, which reminded him of a bishop's hat. Much of the jungle was removed during the colonial era to make room for rubber plantations. Workers relied on Kratom to get through the day's labor, which enhanced the herb's popularity. According to several research, workers who ingested Kratom worked harder than those who smoked marijuana.

Kratom gained popularity after China spread opioids across Asia, and it was shown to be beneficial in the treatment of addiction. Thailand prohibited the use of kratom in Act

486 on 3 August 1943. Local kratom trees have been killed in an attempt to eliminate the plant. The possession of kratom is a capital offence in Thailand, and as a result, more individuals began cultivating it in other areas of Asia, contributing to the herb's growing popularity.

Chapter 9: What Exactly Is Kratom?

Mitragyna Speciosa, often known as Kratom, is a tropical tree that belongs to the same family as coffee plants, and the chemical it produces is regarded as a legitimate psychoactive narcotic in many nations. Because Kratom contains more than 40 recognized active alkaloids, it is quite distinctive and diversified in terms of its effects. The fact that this is one of the most effective natural medications available in Southeast Asia is undeniable. Some of its advantages are as follows:

❖   Euphoria

❖   Relaxation

❖   Pain relief

❖   Vivid waking dreams.

❖   Stimulation

❖   Feelings of empathy

The following are some examples of potential negative consequences:

❖ Nausea and dizziness

❖ Bitter taste

❖ Addiction

❖ Mild depression

❖ Constipation

Although the drug has been related to jaundice in severe cases of addiction, there have been no reports of liver damage associated with regular dosages.

Do Kratoms Contain Opiates or Other Opioids?

With over 40 active alkaloids in kratom, one of the reasons it is so effective for individuals attempting to wean themselves off strong opiates such as heroin is that it contains

Mitragynine, a molecule that has been shown in studies to work as an opioid agonist, which is one of the reasons it is so effective.

Mitragynine

Kratom indeed binds to opioid receptors in the same manner that drugs such as heroin do, but it is nowhere as powerful as heroin in terms of effects. It is believed that the chemical components in Kratom do not produce euphoria.

Following studies, kratom contains a range of phytoalkaloids that do not technically behave as opioid agonists, meaning that if you ingested kratom on the same day that you did a drug test, you would not test positive for the usage of opiates. Even though Kratom contains chemicals that function as opioid agonists, it does not contain any actual opiates. Although kratom includes alkaloids that function as opioid agonists, it is not classified as an opiate under federal law.

How Does Kratom Feel When You Take It?

It is possible to utilize the powdered leaf in quantities ranging from 2–6 grams in place of the normal sedative impact of conventional opiate medications, resulting in an increased sense of energization and focus as opposed to the usual sedative effect.

I would not call taking Kratom in this manner as getting high because it does not provide any high-inducing effects; rather, it can put you in a very peaceful and relaxed state, with a mild euphoric feeling, and even make you chatty.

While the majority of people report feeling good after smoking cannabis, the elevating and euphoric effects aren't as noticeable as they may be. The majority of people would answer that it helps them feel good about themselves. When used in large dosages, it may become highly sedating, comparable to opiates in their conventional form, with the exception that when used frequently, it can cause symptoms such as dysphoria and, most significantly, severe nausea.

Those who take 3 grams or less experience sedation, but those who take more than 6 grams experience sedation. There have been several strains of kratom available from a variety of suppliers that have shown to be beneficial for some people, but they have not proven to be effective for others. Individual tolerance and brain chemistry are also important factors in determining the type of effects that people may experience with kratom. People who are very sensitive to it can get by on as little as 2-3 grams, which is more than enough to improve their mood and put them in a state of heightened energy. Potency is also determined by the quality of the leaf, which is a factor in many cases.

What Kratom Is Capable Of

One of the drug's most important properties is that it works as a partial opioid agonist. For a drug to be labelled an opioid, it must come from the opium poppy plant. In comparison, opioids are medications such as heroin, morphine, oxycodone and hydrocodone that bind to the same receptors found to be present in the brain, spinal cord, digestive system and other areas of the body as do opiates.

A prominent example of an opioid is tramadol, however, kratom is a partial opioid agonist that binds to opioid receptors that are similar, but not identical, to an opioid. They are safe to consume since they have a calming impact on your brain receptors and thus are not addictive. They are not as powerful as opiates.

In this method, 7-hydroxy mitragynine and Mitragynine, which are both more powerful chemicals, attach to receptors in the brain. Mitragynine (7-hydroxy mitragynine) is an opioid agonist having stimulatory properties. Mitragynine includes a small amount of opioid agonists, and mitragynine also has some stimulating properties.

Because the drug is an opioid agonist, it can reduce withdrawal symptoms, discomfort, enhance mood, and relieve muscular tension.

Chapter 10: The Different Kratom Strains and Their Effects

Each Kratom strain is characterized by a distinct color, such as the White vein, the Red vein, or the Green vein, among other characteristics. The identification of the leaves is determined by the stem and vein of the leaf, as well as the colors of the leaves.

When you examine a leaf attentively, you will see that the stem and vein of the leaf have distinct colors.

It is believed that various hues have distinct psychological and biological effects. Distinct colors have different chemical compositions and effects, which are attributed to them. Only the leaves of the kratom plant are harvested, and the fibers are crushed before the stem and vein are removed.

There are numerous distinct kinds of kratom, each of which generates a unique combination of alkaloids that makes it helpful under a variety of different circumstances.

White Vein Kratom

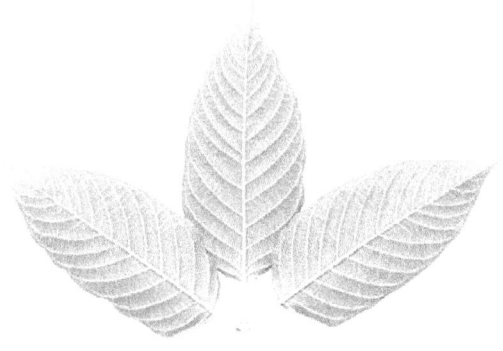

There is little question that the strain has stimulating properties, and it may also be used to improve one's mood when consumed. The advantages are based on a variety of circumstances, including the quality of the product, one's lifestyle, and one's own tolerance. Fundamentally, it is quite stimulating, and it is frequently used in place of coffee to increase feelings of cheerfulness, alertness, and focus.

The vast majority of individuals use it because it increases their motivation, enhances their focus, and gives them more energy to do their tasks.

The use of this strain should not be done too late in the day because it has the potential to make you sleepy. It is standard practice to mix red and white veins to provide a consistent energy level across the body.

Red Vein Kratom

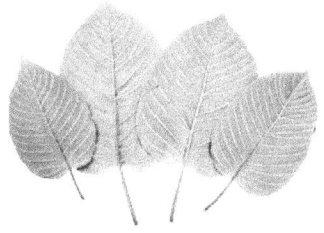

Red Vein Kratom is distinguished by the color of its stem and vein, which are both red. Most customers enjoy this strain, which is why it is one of the best-selling strains on the market today. Having originated in Southeast Asia, it is well-known throughout the region. Compared to green and white veins together, it is significantly more costly.

Finding a dependable supply of red vein leaves is an excellent place to start, especially if you are just beginning started because it has calming benefits and is easy to get by in large quantities. When you meditate, you will experience feelings of well-being and serenity of mind. Using this supplement instead of pain relievers, muscular tension may be relaxed and sleeplessness can be treated without the need for prescription drugs. Its effects and characteristics are diverse, ranging from sedatives like the Red Borneo strain to invigorating strains like the Red Thai.

Green Vein Kratom

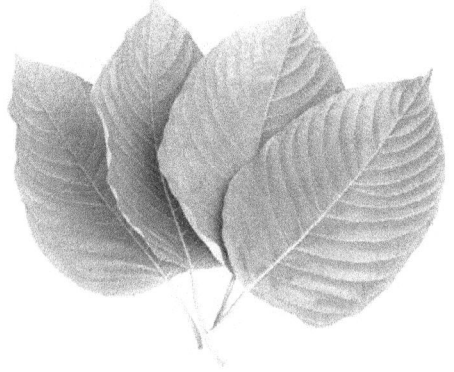

In this category are moderate kratom strains that serve as an energy booster and have the potential to improve your mood. A large number of people have stated that it has assisted them in remaining focused. The treatment can be useful for pain-alleviation, as well as for discomforts induced by other circumstances.

It is possible to combine the green vein kratom with other kratom strains to generate a more mixed flavor with a greater impact by mixing them. It has a well-balanced impact that makes it ideal for dealing with social anxiety. People frequently use this strain for recreational purposes, such as night trips, because it encourages them to converse more and to be happy.

How To Make A Decision Regarding Strain

It is totally up to you to determine which Kratom strain is best for you depending on your requirements and present scenario. When dealing with the same hue, making judgments might be challenging since the impacts vary based on the temperature, the quality of the crop, the location of the crop, and the method of harvesting the crop.

Similarly to how you would not anticipate all red veins to have the same impact, this holds for all other strain colors as well.

A standard set of recommendations for selecting kratom strains and their unique colors are provided in this publication. By purchasing sample packs of kratom powder, you can test the efficacy of any strain and thus choose the one that works best for you. You may also acquire a variety of strains to compare their effects.

Kratom Extract Prepared At Home

Using kratom powder to make kratom extracts at home is a simple, non-conventional approach that can be followed by anybody with a little knowledge of medicine. Powdered kratom is generally the most effective form of kratom to utilize for this approach. Crushed kratom leaves, on the other hand, are also effective. These suggestions will assist you in creating your own.

Electric Stove

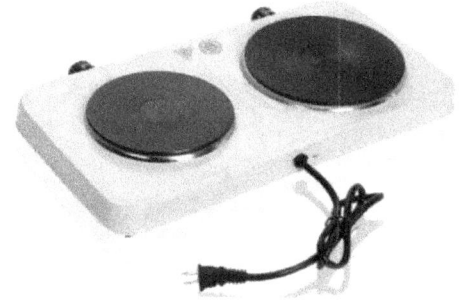

You should use a high setting on an electric stove (7 or 8 on the dial), but you may have to experiment quite a bit with a gas range to obtain the right degree of heat. Open flame/gas stoves are ideal for this experiment, and a decent setting is often approximately 3/4 of the burner's capacity. Maintaining an eye on the boiling water to ensure that it does not burn is important since stoves vary in their performance.

Distilled Water

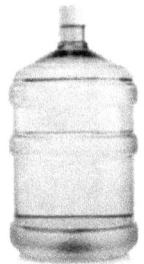

Because this water has no additional minerals, it is often used to make drinking water or bottled water. Because it has no minerals, it is often used in the production of drinking water or bottled water. It is necessary to use one cup of distilled water.

Lemon Juice

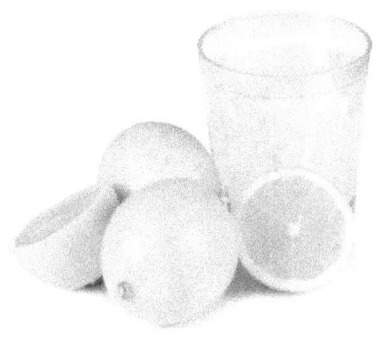

a couple of capfuls of freshly squeezed lemon juice (this will depend on the amount of water and kratom you might be using). This will need the use of two complete caps. Alkaloids are extracted from the Kratom plant when lemon juice is added. Take one or two capsules of lemon juice (the amount of kratom you're taking and the type of water you're using will decide how much you need).

Coffee Grinder

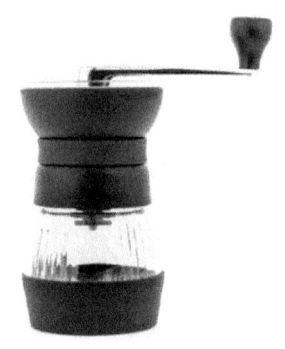

Kratom

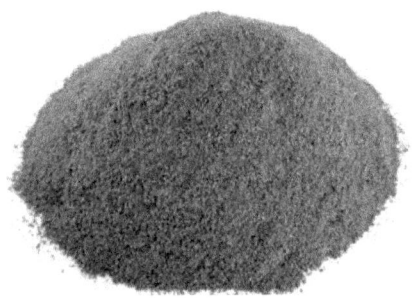

I'll be using 50g of Green Thai Kratom for this recipe. You are able to select any strain that you like from our selection.

Pyrex Stew Pot

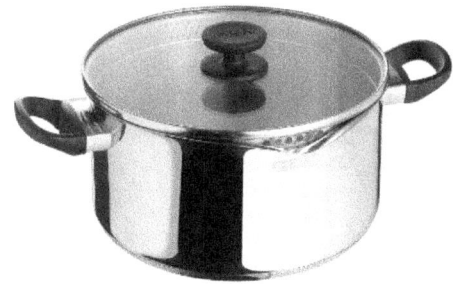

If, for some reason, you do not have a Pyrex pot, you may still make this recipe using a standard pot, but be careful when boiling down the liquid in the last step.

Cheese Cloth

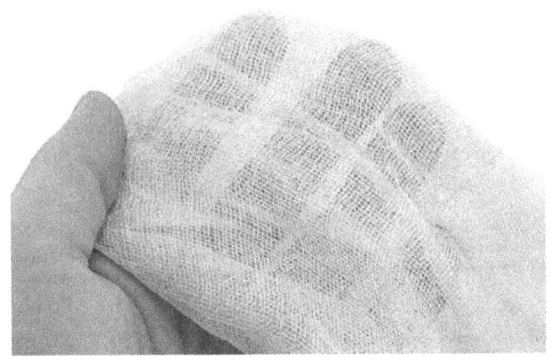

Steps

❖ Two cups of distilled water should be added to the Pyrex saucepan.

❖ Stir in 50g of kratom powder to the water until it is completely dissolved.

❖ Stir in two full caps of lemon juice, followed by one cup of distilled water, until everything is well combined.

❖ Mix the Kratom powder with the lemon juice in the distilled water until thoroughly combined. Cook on high heat (seven or eight) while continually stirring until the water comes to a boil. Make sure that the kratom is thoroughly saturated with water before using it a second time. Stir every 4-8 minutes until it has reduced to a syrupy consistency.

❖ By the time the pot has been boiling for 20 minutes, remove it from the heat to allow it to cool.

❖ After the liquid has cooled, strain it through a cheesecloth or another similar piece of fabric to remove any remaining particles. Pour the liquid into a dish after straining it through the cloth.

❖ After filtering the liquid out of the Kratom, you may put the plant material back into the pot and continue the extraction procedure a second time to get the desired effect. This is done to guarantee that there are no alkaloids left in the plant material after it has been processed.

Both heating the liquid until all of the liquid has evaporated and immediately removing it from heat and allowing it to cool down are acceptable methods for completing this procedure.

To remove the dried Kratom extract from the Pyrex pot, you will need to use a kitchen knife or scraper to carefully cut it out of the container. Pyrex cooking pans were suggested from the beginning of the procedure for the obvious purpose of durability.

Furthermore, the liquid can be reduced until it resembles syrup, after which it can be put onto a ceramic dish and dried in the oven on the lowest temperature setting for several hours. Because the remaining liquid will need to be evaporated, this phase will take longer to complete.

Chapter 11: The Science Behind Opioids and How Do They Work?

Although opioids such as morphine are used for analgesia (pain reduction), let us first review some basic pain perception biology before understanding more about these drugs and how they work to alleviate pain.

Neurons are the building blocks of the brain and nerve cells, and each neuron has a cell body that regulates the activity of the neurons in the brain and nerve cells. Axons are discovered connected to the cell body in addition to the dendrites that are found linked to the cell body. The axon receives signals created inside the cell body, sends them to the dendrites, and then transmits them to other cells in the body.

Axons may also be detected in muscle tissue, which is unusual. Commands must be communicated for them to be controlled.

During neurotransmission, nerves interact with one another by releasing chemical messengers known as neurotransmitters across synaptic connections between neighboring cells. Specific molecules known as receptors are found in the dendrites, and they are responsible for picking up the chemicals produced by the axons.

When your body's receptors are triggered, they transmit instructions to your brain, which is why you have so many different types of receptors. Your body is equipped with thermoreceptors, which alert you whether you are hot or cold. When something is touching you or when you are touching something, you will be able to sense it. Nociceptor receptors, which are sensory receptors that give signals to the brain when stimuli are unpleasant, provide signals to the brain (causing tissue damage).

We tend to think of nociceptors as being restricted to the skin and organ walls, as well as deeper within soft tissues such as muscles, but they are found all over the body.

The nociceptors in your brain communicate with your brain about the pain you just felt when you smashed your finger with a hammer, and your brain responds accordingly. nociceptors are usually thought of as the source of pain, but they are the initial step of a long process that takes place between the nociceptors and the brain. When we are exposed to noxious stimuli, such as touching a hot stove, a primary afferent neuron in the spinal cord delivers an electrical signal to the dorsal root ganglia, which is responsible for pain perception.

Understanding the Process of Opiate Withdrawal

After you begin using opioids, you may find them to be quite enticing at first; but, after using them regularly for at least a few weeks, you will build a resistance to them. To get the same effect, the same dosage of the medication must be taken each time. Physiological dependency on opioids occurs after you have developed tolerance to them and occurs when you no longer require the medication to function, only your neurons and a specific quantity of the substance.

This is an opioid pain reliever that has a down-regulating impact on the central nervous system, which means that once you develop a tolerance, you must ensure that the opioid content in your blood is maintained daily.

In contrast, an opiate withdrawal syndrome characterized by symptoms such as anxiety, diarrhea, depression, sleep difficulties, stomach discomfort, tiredness, and restless leg syndrome might develop. When enough Kratom is used, it is possible to completely eliminate all withdrawal symptoms while also feeling wonderful. Kratom binds to opioid receptors in the brain and has no harmful side effects.

Kratom's Legality

At the moment, there is no regulation of Kratom in the United States by the Drug Enforcement Administration. In 2016, they attempted to prohibit kratom and set a deadline for those who were taking it to make preparations to stop using it, but kratom sellers, American Kratom Associations, and other groups filed a petition against the ban, which was eventually rejected.

In addition to emailing their list and notifying others, they took a variety of other steps to protect themselves.

To get enough signatures on the petition, thousands of citizens wrote to their local officials and signed a petition, which gathered enough signatures. With more than 100,000 signatures, the petition was endorsed by every scientist since there is no proof that the plants are addictive or lethal, but rather that they may be used as a very effective herbal supplement instead. That prompted the Drug Enforcement Administration to lift the ban, which had been in place for several years. The Food and Drug Administration has issued a public statement condemning kratom and claiming that it is possibly lethal.

Although numerous environmental and similar groups have been working diligently in conjunction with many specialists in the field to study the autopsy findings and conclude that kratom was not the cause of their deaths, this has not been the case in recent years.

Kratom Is The Subject Of many Controversies

Thousands of people have learned that kratom may alleviate the symptoms of opiate withdrawal and a variety of other illnesses, and as a result, they are more inclined to select kratom over pharmaceutical medicines. Some individuals believe that kratom is a hazardous chemical because they believe it is substituting one addiction for another, and as a result, it is dangerous; others, on the other hand, believe that it is not dangerous at all.

Kratom for Opiate Addiction Recovery

One glass of wine is more likely to give me a buzz than any amount of kratom, in my opinion. In many states, marijuana, for example, is currently considered lawful. More states will be added shortly. I'm perplexed as to what the issue is here, given that a single shot of marijuana is more potent than any dose of kratom available.

There are moderate herbal variants that help to boost both pain relief and relaxation while also killing opiate cravings as well as anxiety, fear, and enhanced attention. It reminds me of opium pills or coffee that has a trace amount of the drug in it.

Even though I believe the plant is a miracle, I recognize that everyone has the right to their perspective. Since everyone's viewpoint on the world is different, there is no such thing as a neutral point of view; instead, we perceive the world through something known as a lens of reality, which is impacted by the experiences and lessons that we have acquired throughout our lives.

www.ingramcontent.com/pod-product-compliance
Lightning Source LLC
Chambersburg PA
CBHW071336120626
46546CB00002B/580